Stress
and
A Healthy Ticker

Stress
and
A Healthy Ticker

A Psychological Approach to Healing and Preventing Heart Disease

Diana Wisdom, Ph.D.

Writers Club Press
New York   Lincoln   Shanghai

Stress and A Healthy Ticker
A Psychological Approach to Healing and Preventing Heart Disease

Writers Club Press
an imprint of iUniverse, Inc.

For information address:
iUniverse, Inc.
2021 Pine Lake Road, Suite 100
Lincoln, NE 68512
www.iuniverse.com

The information in this book is meant to be useful for people that want to live more fulfilling and healthy lives. While the author is presenting research results, science, and health information concerning cardiac health, it is not the intent of the author to prescribe for or diagnose medical conditions through the use of this book. It may be a useful tool for certain individuals seeking to improve their well-being but it is always prudent to check with one's own health provider before beginning any new treatment approaches. In the event that the information in this book is used without a doctor's approval, you are legally entitled to choose your own treatment approach, but the publisher and author assume no responsibility.

ISBN: 0-595-20414-7

Printed in the United States of America

Epigraph

"When our heart closes in fear, it decreases that flow of life-force energy. It just doesn't get to the cells and tissues in the same way, and we literally starve, because we've cut ourselves off from that larger life force. Every time there is worry, or fear, there is stress, and I've always defined stress as that which is isolating. Anything that takes you out of the sense of connection stresses you."

—Joan Borysenko, Ph.D. in anatomy and cellular biology from Harvard Medical School; Cofounder of the Mind/Body Institute at the Beth Israel Hospital.

"Separation is an optical illusion of consciousness."

—Albert Einstein

"Promoting a sense of connection, community, and intimacy can be healing as well as quieting down the mind enough to experience an inner sense of peace, well-being and connectedness."

—Dean Ornish, M.D. Cardiologist and Founder of the San Francisco Institute of Integrative Medicine

Contents

Acknowledgements

Thank you to my husband, Gabriel Ben, for believing in me.

Thank you to my family and friends for their enduring love, support and encouragement.

Of particular help with this project were Charles Shapiro, Elaine Keyes, Laura Struhl, Ph.D., Stephanie Schneider O.M., Frank Zalman, M.D., Deidra Price, PhD, Gay Parnell, Ph.D., Tyla, Christal Nani, M.A., Lindsey Davidson, Donna Genett, Ph.D., Zev Rosenberg, O.M., Joel Siegal, Richard Levak, Ph.D., patients, and the cardiologists and staff at The San Diego Cardiac Center.

Dr. Dean Ornish, Wayne Dyer, Louise Hay, and Dr. Bernie Siegal have been particularly inspiring in the course of this project.

My thanks to editors Laurie Rosen, Blair Kenney, Charles Shapiro, and Trudie Martineau.

Introduction

Most people are aware these days that heart disease is the number one cause of death in the United States of America and that strokes are the number one cause of disability. Much has been heard over the years about the traditional standard risk factors likely to increase one's odds of developing heart disease, such as obesity, high cholesterol, high blood pressure, cigarette smoking, sedentary lifestyle, and depression. We must examine what is below the surface of these causes to try to understand and offer solutions to the underlying reasons for the current epidemic of heart disease.

Most of the time people have these traditional risk factors for heart disease because they are not coping or living healthily. In my opinion the best medicine for cardiovascular disease is the cultivation of a more loving and compassionate relationship with yourself and those around you. Coping with the stresses of life in a balanced way and developing loving, positive relationships are behaviors highly likely to reduce your risk factor level, whether you are recovering from a cardiac incident or trying to prevent the development of heart problems.

Heart disease is frightening because its course is unpredictable. Physicians can foresee the progress of other illnesses, but heart disease can attack suddenly. Many people feel depressed after their first heart attack. Though remarkable medical advances have been made, a heart attack or heart problem can be a wake-up call.

Most people diagnosed with heart disease feel the need to reevaluate their priorities and change their lifestyles. This reevaluation is a healthy response to a cardiac incident. Stress and A Healthy Ticker is for cardiac patients, their loved ones, and anyone interested in preventing heart disease. In this book you will find recommended behaviors, attitudes, and lifestyles likely to help you cultivate optimal health.

Stress and A Healthy Ticker offers a behavioral-medicine approach to healing heart disease; the connection between stress and heart disease is emphasized. Today mind/body medicine and psychoneuroimmunology are becoming widely accepted models in health care. We are gradually coming to understand the dramatic influence that our thoughts and emotions have on our body. Our mind influences our neurochemicals, hormones, immune system, cardiovascular system, and emotional well-being. This book outlines specific beliefs, attitudes, thoughts, emotions, and behaviors that can enhance or destroy your heart health, and then demonstrates how to make the changes which may reduce your chances of early death or disability due to heart disease.

The spiritual undertones in this book are not intended to promote any particular religious orientation; the focus is rather to present practical suggestions that are likely to improve your condition of health and happiness. Learning to change our internal approach to life is not a simple task; it is an ongoing process for a lifetime. Through learning and self-discipline we can repair our hearts, calm our minds, and dramatically improve our quality of life. Every little step any of us make in this direction is worthwhile. My personal and professional aim is to always become a more compassionate, calm, loving, playful, and productive person. This book is my effort to share some of what I've learned in my studies, research, practice, and personal journey.

When we create a society of people who are less reactive and more loving, we will have less heart disease and more peace internally and externally. My hope is that you will use this information toward your own healing.

Chapter One

The Heart Attack

"When we long for life without difficulties, remember that oaks grow strong in contrary winds, and diamonds are made under pressure."

—Peter Marshall

April 3, 11:45 P.M.

It's hard to breathe. My heart feels as if it's beating in my throat. I've been sitting in the hospital waiting room for what seems like hours while Dad has open-heart surgery after his heart attack. Time seems to have stopped. I'm terrified, watching the clock and wondering if the batteries are running down because the hands are moving so slowly. My own heart feels as if it's going to jump out of my chest. I wish Mom were here. I'm just his daughter. "Little Alice," he used to call me.

Mrs. Orangey, his neighbor, was at the hospital when I arrived. She found him lying on the kitchen floor in his house. His bathrobe had come open when he fell, so Mrs. Orangey discovered him sprawled on his back with his body exposed. I didn't appreciate Mrs. Orangey telling me all these details. Dad's always been so private and in control that I know he wouldn't want me to hear this.

I listened, because I didn't know what else to do and I felt numb, but I really wanted to wring her neck and scream "Just tell me if he's going to be okay!"

Dad was supposed to pick her up for their weekly bridge game. When he didn't arrive she got worried. Dad usually runs late, but he always shows up less than a half hour from the appointed time. When he hadn't shown, Mrs. Orangey had her long-awaited opportunity to use her emergency spare key to Dad's place.

I don't know why I have to be so down on her. Who knows what would have happened if she hadn't gone looking for him? It's just that she really gets on my nerves, trying so hard to be nice. She found him and called 911 and then called me…Dad's still in surgery. The doctor said he had a myocardial infarction, so they had to open him up. I'm not sure what it all means, but it's terrifying to think of Dad in there with his chest opened up and his heart exposed. So many complications can arise once a person is opened up. That I know. I'm worried, but not really surprised. In a way, this has been a long time in coming. He wouldn't take good care of himself.

April 4, 12:30 A.M.

I can't look at these sickly green walls anymore. When is someone going to come and tell me something? I finally told Mrs. Orangey to go home. It was a strain to have her here, so I'm better off waiting alone. I can hear myself think better—not that I'm having any profound thoughts. If anything, I'm driving myself crazy with worry. She probably would've been a good distraction, but I didn't want to have to make idle conversation and worry about her being upset. Yeah, I know she means well.

April 4, 3:30 A.M.

Dad made it through the surgery okay. I'm exhausted, but I can't sleep for the thoughts swimming in my head. I almost lost Dad today. He's my one remaining parent, and I don't even know him well. The thought that I almost lost him keeps echoing in my mind. I tell myself I'll spend more time with him when he feels better.

Now maybe he'll start taking better care of himself. Maybe. I wonder if heart problems run in families. Scary thought. I'll have to learn what I can do to help Dad get well—and stay healthy myself.

I wish I could sleep.

April 4, 10:15 P.M.

It was hard to focus on my job today because I was worrying about Dad. He looked so pale and tired; I was frightened. Yet he complained about staying in the hospital. The doctor says he needs to stay there a couple more days before I take him home. It's hard to see Dad like this, and not be able to help him or even know how to comfort him. We don't talk much about feelings, so times like this are awkward between us; I don't know what to say. I'm afraid that if I fuss over him too much, he'll get mad.

I don't want to do anything to upset him or rock the boat in any way. It's pretty pathetic that I'm so worried about my own dad getting mad at me that I don't even know how to help him. Ridiculous.

April 5, 7:30 P.M.

Dad was very groggy and out of it. Mrs. Orangey came by to visit, all warm and huggy, inviting me over to dinner. I wish I could accept her gestures, but I feel frozen and unfriendly around her. I just want to be alone to figure out about Dad and me.

What is she to Dad anyway—just a neighbor and a bridge partner? Fat chance! She's had her eye on him ever since Mom died, and she sees this as an opportunity to make her move. He's going to be vulnerable for a bit, and I don't appreciate her closing in for the kill.

Okay, maybe I'm being too harsh. She seems to care, but I have a hard time letting her get close to me, and I can't imagine that Dad's comfortable with her hovering around him. He's never liked people fussing over him. He's always been very independent and in control. Both of us asked how he felt. "I'm fine," he kept saying. "Tired, but fine. Stop asking me!"

He taught me that weakness and dependency were bad, but now we have a whole different ball game. He's flat on his back and seems really depressed. I hate not knowing what to do for him.

Ever since Mom died he's been even more distant, telling me that I shouldn't trust anyone and that you have to make your own way in life and not lean on other people. Now that he needs to lean on me, he won't know how, and I won't know what to do. He seems so far away. I wish we were more relaxed with each other instead of so strained and guarded.

April 6, 2:30 A.M.

I can't sleep again. It's always been a constant problem, but now I'm worse than ever, lying in bed, gripped with fears that Dad won't survive. This time, instead of just lying awake, I looked up heart disease on the Internet. I found a report that Americans have a higher chance of dying of heart disease than of anything else.

It's the number one cause of death in industrialized countries, and just as many women die as men. Serious heart problems are becoming more common among people between thirty-five and fifty, and heart problems might be genetic. That's scary.

They list things that people can do to help prevent heart disease, so Dad and I had better pay attention.

April 6, 6:00 P.M.

I spent the early morning with Dad. Awkward. Neither of us knew what to say to each other. Have we ever? No wonder I don't spend more time with him; I always feel as if I don't measure up to his expectations. Sometimes I'm mad and frustrated and just want to stay away, and other times I want his approval. Because of his heart attack, my longing for his approval has intensified. What if I lose him forever and he's never been proud of me?

I'll learn as much as I can about how to prevent and recover from heart disease so I can support him in a way he'll appreciate. No touchy-feely stuff—just information. That way I won't get mushy with Dad, and I won't have time to hang around him, nervously checking to see if he's okay and trying to make conversation.

Mrs. Orangey has been like a mother hen, and I can tell he doesn't like it from her, so why would he like it from me? Maybe I can rescue him from her by telling her that he is tired and shouldn't have too many visitors. She seems nice enough, but she bugs me.

Doctor's Notepad

Certain behavior patterns place us at a higher risk than usual for developing heart disease. These behaviors are characteristic of the type A personality. Substantial research over the past ten years has determined that not the drive to achieve, but a tendency toward chronic hostility, irritability, distrust, and consequent social isolation with a lack of close, loving relationships places a person at a high risk of developing heart disease.

This behavior pattern is common in Western societies, especially the United States. Heart disease is the number one cause of death in the United States, and stroke is the number one cause of disability.

The term "coronary-prone behavior pattern" is used to describe these tendencies. CPBP is a more optimistic term than "type A personality" in that it is easier to change a behavior pattern than a whole personality.

People with CPBP exhibit the following characteristics:

- Emotional reactivity. They become angry quickly and harbor feelings of hostility.
- Fierce independence and need to be in control. They are leaders and have difficulty "going with the flow."
- Difficulty with intimacy. They fear open, honest self-disclosure of thoughts and feelings.
- Time urgency. They are usually in a hurry and, for example, hate waiting in lines.
- Mistrust of other people.
- Underlying feelings of depression and isolation.

Cardiac incidents can traumatize the patient and the family. People with CPBP are uncomfortable if they are vulnerable or needy, and they have difficulties in close relationships. They need to be in charge. The family needs to know how best to be helpful and supportive to the patient. Alice and her father both demonstrate CPBP. She is just as uncomfortable with intimacy as he is, so she decides to keep busy learning about heart disease as a way to avoid spending time with him. Alice is right to learn about her father's disease, but she unintentionally uses her research to distance herself from her father, just as other people with CPBP use work, household chores, or any of the endless tasks of life as excuses to avoid spending quality time with their loved ones. Patients frequently experience depression from a combination of factors after heart procedures. The physical trauma experienced by the body can cause a patient to withdraw as a useful defensive action while the body is healing. The patient might be distressed by a feeling of loss of control over his body or his destiny. Underlying depression that the individual had previously been able to ignore by staying busy might surface now that he is unable to distract himself.

Patients depressed after heart procedures should discuss these feelings with a caring friend or mental health professional. In most cases the depression will lift in time, unless an underlying depression preceded the cardiac incident. If so, the depression might grow worse after the heart procedure, and specific treatment for depression could be necessary for a full recovery. Anti-depressant medication can be very helpful in reducing symptoms of depression, especially if medication is combined with a therapy that focuses on changing the thoughts and behaviors that reinforce the depression.

Symptoms Of Depression
(National Institute of Mental Health—NIMH)

- Persistent sad, anxious, or "empty" mood
- Feelings of hopelessness, pessimism
- Feelings of guilt, worthlessness, helplessness
- Loss of interest or pleasure in hobbies and activities that were once enjoyed, including sex
- Decreased energy, fatigue, being "slowed down"
- Difficulty concentrating, remembering, making decisions
- Insomnia, early-morning awakening, or oversleeping
- Appetite and/or weight changes
- Thoughts of death or suicide, or suicide attempts
- Restlessness, irritability

If five or more of these symptoms are present every day for at least two weeks and interfere with routine daily activities such as work, self-care, and childcare of social life, seek an evaluation for depression.

Chapter Two

The Family Physician: Traditional Perspectives on Heart Disease

"People are much more likely to choose life-enhancing behaviors than self-destructive ones when they feel loved and cared for."

—Dean Ornish, M.D., cardiologist, researcher, and author.

April 6, 9:00 A.M.

I stopped in for a brief visit with Dad after work. He still seems terribly tired. He says that his doctor wants him to participate in the cardiac rehab program before and after he leaves the hospital, but he has no interest in it. He just complains that he's tired and wants to go home.

It hurts to see him like this.

I made several appointments with heart specialists today. I'm behind on my quotas at work, but I'll make them up by the end of the month. I am excited about talking to different experts to learn more about preventing heart disease and helping Dad in his recovery.

I felt like I should've stayed with Dad longer today, but I wanted to come home and get some questions ready for interviews with doctors. He didn't seem to mind my leaving.

April 7, 10:00 A.M.

I met with Dr. Frank, our family doctor, this morning. I've always liked him and felt comfortable with him. He was very sympathetic about Dad and asked how he could help. I told him about my research project and asked him what heart disease is. He said that coronary disease is almost always related to problems with the arteries that supply blood and oxygen to the heart muscle and told me about the different types of heart disease.

I said I'm most interested in how to prevent and recover from heart disease, and he replied that the key is reducing the standard risk factors. I tried to take careful notes, but I couldn't listen and write at the same time. I was afraid I would miss something important. Next time maybe I'll listen as carefully as I can, jot down major points, and later fill in the notes about the meeting.

I think I got all of the standard risk factors: cigarette smoking, high cholesterol, obesity, hypertension, sedentary lifestyle, and stress. He said that stress can change the body's chemistry, and over time this change in chemistry can cause great wear and tear on the cardiovascular system.

I asked about the stress component—life is stressful, and nobody can avoid life—he recommended the name and phone number of a cardiologist and a psychologist whom I could interview for more details. Dr. Frank also suggested that I go to Dad's cardiac rehab program with him to check out the family part and whatever classes they will let me attend. Maybe, but I really don't know how I'd find the time, and besides, I've never liked group things. Maybe I'm like Dad.

He said Dad could use emotional support—sounds like a good idea, but what I need is a how-to manual for my particular dad. How can I give him emotional support when he won't let me close, trained me not to expect or want closeness, and practically taught me that it's a sign of weakness?

Now I'm whining. Dr. Frank asked me to tell Dad "Hello" for him, and said that he would give him a call to check on him. That was nice.

April 7, 6:30 P.M.

I'm sitting in the backyard of Dad's house, watching dusk meet the fall evening. A crisp, light breeze with a scent of lavender honeysuckle is floating in the air. Pine needles are rustling. I came here to feel close to Dad, because he's on my mind all the time. Nagging, obsessive, unproductive thoughts of work buzz in my head, distracting me only momentarily from my worries about Dad. I don't know how I'd cope with losing him. Then I get mad at myself for having such terrible thoughts and letting awkwardness and fear get in the way of knowing him while I still have the chance.

Thinking about everything that I need to do makes me dizzy. I can't relax.

I wish Dad was here now, and I feel guilty that I haven't spent more time with him. This research project will give us something to talk about, and all my effort will show him how much I care about him. He respects accomplishments, so I'll teach him what I learn, and I hope it'll bring us closer. Or am I just kidding myself?

Why am I crying? What an idiot! God, if you exist, could you please help my dad? I'm ridiculous, sitting here pretending to pray when I don't even know how to, and would God listen anyway? I clench my fists, and I can feel the fingernails dig into my palm. I don't care. Boy, am I in sad shape!

April 8, 5:00 P.M.

I stopped by to see Dad at the hospital tonight. I wanted to visit him before his dinner came so I'd have a convenient excuse to leave. The nurses kept me waiting outside his room for twenty minutes while they did some procedure. I was so mad when I kept telling them that I was his daughter and should be allowed to go in, but it didn't seem to matter to them. Protocol overrode human considerations. Maybe he'd have wanted me in there. That might have been a chance to offer him emotional support. Easy to say, now that I missed the chance.

Anyway, I hate waiting, especially when I don't have anything to do. Writing about my frustration is at least better than doing nothing.

April 8, 5:15 P.M.

Now I'm feeling bad for being so impatient while waiting for Dad. I'm selfish. It's just that I hate feeling that I'm wasting my time when I could be doing other things.

April 8, 10:00 P.M.

Dad seemed happy to see me today. That felt good. He *said* he was okay, but he looked terrible, so I didn't want to push it. I told him about my research project; I didn't know what else to talk about. He wasn't very enthusiastic, saying he was worried that it would be time-consuming and expensive to interview all sorts of health professionals. I told him I was meeting with doctors for free. At first he didn't seem to believe me, and then he seemed concerned about my wasting their time! I can't win with him, but then I'm not sure he's ever been supportive of any of my ideas.

When they brought in his dinner tray the nurse asked if I'd like to join him, saying that she could bring me a tray. I felt like I should stay, but I was uncomfortable because I couldn't tell if Dad really wanted me to or not. Anyway, I needed to go home and get my questions ready for tomorrow's interviews. Still, I feel badly about leaving him. I am hopeful this will all work out. Dad will find the information helpful, he'll appreciate all my efforts, and he will get well, and we'll have lots more time together.

April 9, 5:00 A.M.

I had disturbing dreams, filled with fears and doubts about whether I can really help Dad with this research project. In one dream Mom was here telling me to spend more time with Dad. "He needs you more than information," she said. Her face was soft and encouraging. I was a little girl, and she was sitting on the edge of my bed, tucking me in for the night, as she did in my favorite memories. If only Mom were here. I woke up with my stomach aching—a familiar gnawing feeling of insecurity.

Doctor's Notepad

Alice learns about the standard risk factors for heart disease: cigarette smoking, high cholesterol, obesity, hypertension, sedentary lifestyle, and chronic stress. Genetic factors aside, chronic stress might be the most important risk factor and the main culprit in the development of heart disease. Smoking, over-eating, high cholesterol, high blood pressure, depression, and sedentary lifestyle all contribute to the risk of heart disease. They are all unhealthy attempts to cope with stress. Better methods of coping with daily challenges can help you manage stress and improve your health.

Through her diary, Alice shows us the kind of thinking, belief system, and emotions common to people who display CPBP. As Alice interviews different medical experts about how to prevent heart disease, she slowly realizes that she has CPBP. She begins to reevaluate her life and tries to make the changes suggested by the doctors. She goes through a gradual transformation and demonstrates how adopting different attitudes and behaviors can help save one's life.

People with CPBP are most at risk for developing cardiac illness. Changing one's lifestyle is not easy, but making the recommended changes is possible. You can dramatically improve the quality of your life.

Coronary heart disease (CHD)—the number one cause of death in most Western countries—involves a disorder of the arteries that supply blood to the heart muscle. Types of coronary heart disease include angina pectoris, myocardial infarction, ischemic cardiomyopathy, and sudden cardiac death. Also, CHD often results from arteriosclerosis: hardening or blocking of the arteries.

The arteries of a person with arteriosclerosis are lined with fatty cholesterol deposits and plaque, which slow the delivery of blood to the heart. Angina pectoris involves brief periodic attacks of chest pain caused by insufficient delivery of blood to the heart. A myocardial infarction is a heart attack which occurs when the lack of blood and oxygen is so severe that part of the heart muscle actually dies. Sudden cardiac death happens when a person dies a short time after an unexpected onset of symptoms. Ischemic cardiomyopathy refers to a malfunction of the heart muscle without any evident medical cause.

Symptoms of cardiac illness or a heart attack include chest discomfort (can be in the center of the chest or your upper back). It can last a few minutes or more, or go away and come back. It can feel like pressure, squeezing, pain, or ache. Symptoms may include pain, ache, and pressure in arms, jaw, neck or stomach. Shortness of breath, cold sweats, nausea or light headedness can also indicate cardiac illness. When a person has one or more of these signs for five minutes or longer, they should not hesitate to either call 9-1-1 or have someone else drive them to a nearby hospital. Early intervention can make a world of difference in one's chances of survival and optimal recovery.

Individuals with depression seem to be more vulnerable than others to ischemic heart disease. Depression usually involves feelings of sadness, hurt, frustration, and anger that are not expressed. Holding in painful emotions over long periods of time can cause physical stress to the cardiovascular system.

The approach an individual takes toward the challenges of life helps determine the degree of wear and tear that the body suffers. For instance, our physiological response to stress is an increase in adrenalin, epinephrine, or norepinephrine0151which causes a thickening of the blood, increased heart rate, vascular constriction, and higher blood pressure.

Stress can be caused by physical, mental, or emotional pressures. The physiological stress response was designed to support our primitive fight-or-flight needs. During a physiological stress response the body simultaneously prepares to flee and to attack. Internal messages of stress cause our blood to thicken, and if one is physically wounded the vascular system constricts.

The fight-or-flight response is a primitive coping mechanism that has been wired into our brains. The daily stressors in today's society are not likely to require this intense physiological reaction. When the chemicals aroused by stress surge within the body, the body assumes that this is a life-or-death situation, so it responds by increasing chemicals like adrenaline, which cause the blood to thicken to lessen the risk of bleeding to death. The breathing becomes rapid and shallow, and the heart beats faster. Less oxygen and blood reach the heart, and the blood pressure increases.

If a person responds many times a day to relatively small stressors or irritations with this fight-or-flight stress response, his cardiovascular system will wear out sooner, rather than later.

A new study by Catherine Stoney, PhD, at Ohio State University found that short periods of psychological stress can cause the body to take longer to clear heart damaging fats from the bloodstream. It seems that during stress, fat is not metabolized as quickly or efficiently. This finding offers just one of the reasons why stress has been linked to heart disease.

The Coronary-Prone Behavior Pattern includes strong emotional reactions to relatively minor stressors, time urgency, and chronic mistrust of other people. People who have CPBP trigger the fight-or-flight chemical reactions in their body many times a day. A healthier psychological approach to life is required if we are to reduce our chances of prematurely damaging our heart.

Depression, anxiety, time-urgency, chronic irritability or hostility can be caused by many factors. Three common causes are biochemical imbalances in the brain and unhealthy thinking and behavior patterns. Medications for depression, anxiety, and mood stabilization can be life changing for people who are suffering with C.P.B.P. and other destructive behavior patterns. These psychotropic medications can help the person calm down and be motivated to work on changing their thinking, reactivity, and behavior patterns. Little gold nuggets that can help you begin to make these changes are sprinkled throughout this book.

Chapter Three

The Cardiologist: Stress and The Coronary Prone Behavior Pattern

"Everyone talks about heart disease being linked to negative emotions, such as anger, depression, and so on. But I view all these internal vascular changes as hidden forms of communication, like blushing. The vascular changes are the language of the heart."

—James J. Lynch, Ph.D., professor of psychiatry, University of Maryland Medical School

April 9, 7:00 A.M.

I'm nervous about meeting with the cardiologist today. I hope he doesn't think my questions are dumb.

April 9, 4:00 P.M.

The morning meeting with Dad's cardiologist, Dr. James, seemed to go well. It was kind of him to take time to talk with me. He gave me a tour of the office and showed me the equipment used for diagnosis and treatment. It was impressive, but I didn't understand most of the complicated high-tech stuff. He tried to explain what the machines were used for, but I got lost in the terminology.

He said Dad's doing okay, and it's normal for patients to feel tired, disoriented, and depressed after having open-heart surgery. He seemed to think it was a good idea for me to learn about heart disease. I hope he wasn't just humoring me, but it didn't seem that way.

He focused on stress as a risk factor in heart disease, just as Dr. Frank had. Dr. James believes that managing stress well is important to prevention and recovery. He mentioned that cardiac illness is really tough on the patients, because it can strike at any time without warning, and then they have to live the rest of their life dealing with the results.

He gave me the name of a psychologist and a sociologist I can contact, and also recommended a stress management specialist in Dad's cardiac rehab program at the hospital. Dad had told Dr. James he didn't want to participate in the cardiac rehab, so the doctor asked me to encourage him any way I can.

He told me about the different types of heart disease, but focused on coronary artery disease, the most common illness. Smoking is worse for the heart than anything else. He explained some interesting details I never knew before about how smoking contributes to heart disease, but I didn't write them down because I was too panicked about the fact that I am a social smoker. I didn't have the nerve to ask him how dangerous it is to smoke only occasionally, like I do. Maybe I'm too worried about what people think. He must know that people smoke.

I do lose details if I don't write them down, but I get flustered and embarrassed if I try to act like a secretary, so I'm continuing to absorb the information during the meeting and write it down afterward.

Dr. James talked about controlling high blood pressure, cholesterol, and nutrition, then said he doesn't understand why, even though we know that obesity contributes to most diseases, most of us Americans keep getting heavier all the time. I need to get back to the gym. But there's always something else to do—getting gas in the car, going to the dry cleaners, the bank, the market, whatever...

I feel down. Friends have called, but I haven't wanted to call them back. I don't feel as if they can relate to my problems. Also, I'm extremely irritable and better off staying away from people so I don't alienate them. So I stay busy with this project and work when I can, although my heart's just not in my job these days. Selling advertising for the radio station just doesn't seem as important as figuring this heart disease thing out. Maybe I am nervous because the CPBP that the doctors keep describing fits Dad and me! I feel a little freaked.

Dad had a heart attack because a blood clot formed inside an artery and interrupted the blood flow to that area of the heart, so part of that heart muscle died. Awful! But it is interesting to understand what actually happened. He had the attack on his and mom's wedding anniversary. Could that have had anything to do with it?

I've learned that symptoms of a heart attack include a pressure or tightness in the chest, sometimes with a burning sensation in the arm, jaw, shoulder or shoulder blades; also fatigue, fainting, sudden sweating, nausea, and shortness of breath. My breath is short right now as I'm writing this. The most common symptom among women is sharp pain in the chest area, which I get a lot when I'm stressed. Dr. James said that a person usually has more than one of these symptoms at a time.

It's important for people not to ignore their symptoms, especially if they have two or more of them. Dad's always been so tough; he would push past however his body felt. I thought being tough was a good thing, but if he had listened to his body, maybe he wouldn't have had a heart attack.

Dr. James said the earlier people come in for help with a cardiac problem, the better chance he has of being able to help them. I asked if he thought it would be possible for a person with CPBP to change and reduce his risk, and he answered, "When people are motivated enough, anything is possible."

He also said he believes most people with CPBP suffer from depression and anxiety, and counseling and medication can help them cope in new ways. I asked if he refers patients to counseling or suggests antidepressant medications, but he admitted that he rarely does so. As a technician, he focuses on his specialty of the mechanics of the cardiovascular system. He is not trained to recognize emotional problems, and mentions them only when they're extremely obvious. I doubt if Dad would go to a counselor, even if the doctor recommended one.

Dr. James was really forthcoming. He said one of his patients cried during exams, and he referred her to a psychologist. Maybe when you know you're really good at one thing you can afford to be real about your weaknesses.

He offered to have a friend of his call me—a doctor who had a heart attack and has since changed himself and his lifestyle quite a bit. He said his friend would probably enjoy talking with me. That was very kind of him, or was it just a good way to get rid of me? He gave me several names and phone numbers.

April 9, 10:00 P.M.

I feel very anxious. The more I learn, the more worried I get. What if Dad has another heart attack and dies? What if I have a heart attack twenty years from now? What if Dad has no interest in the information, and it doesn't help me to connect with him, and I continue to feel so lost? I guess I'm just feeling sorry for myself. Things aren't so bad.

What a joke! As I learn how stress causes heart disease, I get even more stressed. I need to apply to myself what I'm learning in regard to preventing this disease instead of just getting more worried and feeling as if I'm doomed.

April 10, 8:00 A.M.

I woke up anxious and decided to start working on changing my lifestyle. I have to practice what I'm going to preach. If I want to get Dad moving his body, I've got to do it, too. I worked out early this morning, but I was keyed up, and my chest felt so tight I had difficulty breathing.

Even getting to the gym was stressful because of heavy traffic. Another car cut me off, honking and honking at me, scaring me half to death. I got so mad my blood was boiling. I don't need the stress of stupid, inconsiderate drivers when I'm in the middle of driving to the gym in order to exercise to reduce my stress. Of course now I'm mad at myself for getting mad. I want to make my world safe and peaceful, but there's no way I can. I feel defeated this morning.

I thought about visiting Dad at lunch today, but I think I'll wait until I've done more on my research project. Maybe tomorrow I'll have some answers, and that'll give us something to talk about. Today I'll call him instead and try to sound cheerful.

April 10, 11:55 P.M.

I spent too much time on my computer, so it was too late to call Dad. Guilty feeling. I will definitely make it a priority to visit him tomorrow. I hope he isn't mad at me. The time just disappears when I'm on-line. That must be why they call it "cyberspace."

I answered several E-mails after deleting a bunch of spam. It's easier to E-mail friends than to talk to them on the phone—takes less energy and is more efficient. Of course it's a more distant kind of connection, but I feel like being alone.

I'm overwhelmed. I promised myself that I'd keep notes on these interviews, but I keep writing about how I feel. People say it's important to let yourself feel your emotions. I'm not sure I see why, because it just sucks energy out of me and interferes with my productivity.

The Cardiologist: Stress and The Coronary Prone Behavior Pattern

Doctor's Notepad

Alice is learning more about the physical and psychological aspects of the CPBP lifestyle. Coronary-Prone Behavior Pattern is a stressful lifestyle. When a human being senses a threat or feels under attack, certain parts of her nervous system are activated. Her body responds by increasing blood supply to the heart and skeletal muscles, and decreasing blood to the skin and other organs.

When the body is under stress, the adrenal cortex releases hormones which are similar to cortisone. Research has shown that excessive cortisone can lead to an increase in blockages of the coronary arteries; so in essence, a person who is frequently stressed might develop an excess of cortisone in the body, which can result in the body overdosing on its own hormones.

Over time, the excess of these chemicals secreted into the system creates layers of plaque in the arteries. The plaque constricts blood circulation and flow, making the heart and entire vascular system vulnerable to cardiac problems. Hostility, chronic overwork, too much stress, and exhaustion can trigger this chemical stress response in the body and predispose one to develop cardiac illness.

While most cardiologists genuinely care about their patients, they are usually focused on their highly sophisticated medical responsibilities and don't have the time nor the training to address the emotional, psychological, or lifestyle aspects of treatment. Cardiology is a complex specialty which demands much attention to detail. Specialists must maintain an exceptionally high level of skill and continually update their knowledge through education and research.

They cannot be expected to be counselors and psychologists, in addition to their medical expertise. Because behavioral medicine is becoming recognized as a helpful adjunct in treating and preventing cardiac and vascular diseases, more cardiology offices are hiring nurses and other health professionals to teach and advocate healthy lifestyle changes to patients.

Cigarette smoking is clearly associated with heart attacks. Nicotine creates an eighty-four percent increase in adrenalin secretion. The Coronary-Prone Behavior Pattern includes tendencies toward anxiety, chronic worry, and depression, and individuals who tend to be anxious or depressed are more likely than others to smoke because nicotine has anti-anxiety and antidepressant effects. As a matter of fact, nicotine was originally used as a tranquilizer for elephants.

As well as being unhealthy, nicotine is highly addictive, since the relaxing and energizing benefits of nicotine only last for about twenty seconds before the smoker needs another dose. Even occasional smoking is harmful to one's health. Smoking is like playing with a loaded gun.

When a person is chronically depressed, anxious, worried, or excessively drawn toward mind altering chemicals (including adrenaline), the causes of the imbalance need to be assessed. The mind/body approach suggests looking at the combination of lifestyle, thought patterns, and biochemistry. There are many avenues for adjusting biochemistry—including dietary and exercise changes, thought pattern changes, herbs, medication, and acupuncture—to name a few.

Chronic emotional stress can create changes in biochemistry and ultimately bring on a heart attack, especially if the stress has been longstanding. The highest number of heart attacks occurs on Monday morning at nine o'clock. Experts hypothesize that this happens because people are returning to jobs they do not enjoy, or jobs they find stressful. A surge of emotion—either depression or excitement—is accompanied by a surge in adrenalin, which can precipitate a heart attack.

Healthy coping skills and balanced lifestyles are the antidote for our epidemic of heart disease. Most people are capable of learning healthy coping skills, which promote a more enjoyable quality of life. Many people wait until they have had a frightening cardiac incident before they make the changes that will help save their life. I say "Why wait?" Use the information in this book to start making these changes now!

Chapter Four

The Sociologist: Intimacy, Loneliness, and the Benefit of Community

"A lot of what we see as disease states is a starvation for love and connection."

—Harvey Zarren, M.D., board-certified cardiologist and associate professor of clinical medicine at the Tufts University School of Medicine.

April 11, 6:00 P.M.

I tried to make up for lost time at work today, but I had a bad day. I got impatient with my assistant and some customers. Jane walked up to my desk and said, "Good morning. Where have you been?" I was irritated—just didn't feel like having to explain myself. I don't know if she noticed or not. It's hard enough to try to concentrate and get some work done.

My mind keeps going back to what I could be doing for Dad. I feel helpless and scared. There's not much I can do about it, so I just have to push my fears away and keep going to catch up and meet my quota. I don't want to have to explain about Dad to Jane or anyone else. I've got to stay busy and keep my mind on my job.

April 11, 10:00 P.M.

There's not enough time in the day to do everything. Recently my energy has gone up and down even more than usual, so I have to wait until I feel energetic and then get as much done as I can. It's hard to be nice to people who want to talk to me about stuff that doesn't have anything to do with what I'm trying to accomplish, then I feel bad and worry that I was too short with them.

Jill and Rachel have been calling, wanting to get together, and asking why they haven't heard from me. I don't want to call them back—don't feel as if anyone can really understand how I feel about Dad's heart attack.

Unless you've been there, you can't know what it's really like. I love him and need him, but I don't feel comfortable with him. I'm scared at the thought of losing him, and I'm mad at him. There, I said it!

April 11, 10:30 P.M.

I just got off the phone with Jill. She really is a good friend. I told her I'm very busy right now and promised I'd call her soon to make plans. I need to wait till I finish this project for Dad and then catch up on my quotas at work. I'm nervous because I'll visit Dad tomorrow, and he'll be going home soon to live alone. I made an appointment with a sociologist for tomorrow, also, so it'll be a busy day.

April 12, 3:00 P.M.

I'm sitting in a pretty restaurant outdoors on the oceanfront after having lunch with Dr. Judy, the sociologist. It's beautiful here, so why don't I come more often? I'll jot down some notes while they're fresh in my mind.

I liked her. She said modern life has become increasingly complicated. The Information Age is overwhelming to many people, and in Western societies—where accomplishment and achievement are expected—the pressure on everyone has increased dramatically. She mentioned faxes and E-mail as examples of the inventions that push us to want instant answers in contrast to snail mail, the old-fashioned letter that takes at least a day to arrive.

She said that while heart disease is reported as the number one cause of death in the United States, loneliness is the number one disease. People are less connected to each other and to their communities, so more people are socially isolated. I feel isolated, but then I feel guilty because it's not as if I don't have opportunities to socialize. I do. Why don't I want to see my friends?

I don't, because I'm so focused on my own projects: my job, my new research project, and so on. What's wrong with that? Nothing in itself, I guess, but she said societies that have strong, close communities have much less heart disease. I never thought about a relationship between diseases of the heart and relationships with people. It's kind of poetic.

She said that traditionally, women have been good at creating relationships and helping communities, but now that women are busy out in the work world, they don't have as much time or energy to tend the home fires, and this change has weakened the social fabric of our culture. She wasn't saying that women should stay home; she was just trying to explain that women are expected to nurture the family and the community and that with more and more women working "the social fabric is fraying."

She said that Greece and Italy are good examples of cultures with "a close-knit cultural fabric." Greeks and Italians talk about their feelings—their dreams, fears, and spiritual beliefs. She laughed and said that for a long time we thought their high consumption of olive oil was the reason they had much less heart disease than we do, but now she believes the reason is the close nurturing communities that are the fabric of their culture.

Our culture worships achievement, so we get isolated as we try to reach our goals. We tell ourselves that when we accomplish such and such, we'll start spending more time with friends and family. I can see that we tend to focus on what's next, rather than looking at what we've already accomplished and how far we've come. We never feel as if we can relax and enjoy ourselves and our loved ones.

What can I do about it? Since Dad's been sick, I've been trying to help him, and I've neglected my friends. I must admit I do feel lonely, but I just can't relax until I've gotten a certain amount done. Am I fooling myself? Will I be able to relax even then?

Dr. Judy said that people long for close relationships, meaning, and a sense of belonging. We need to start building stronger, healthier communities that encourage children in the direction of social interdependence. I think she's right.

She gave the analogy of redwood trees. Redwoods are huge, magnificent trees, but they have very shallow roots, like Americans who move from community to community, more now than ever before.

Each redwood tree interweaves its roots with those of the neighboring trees, thereby creating a supportive infrastructure—a community of trees. This infrastructure protects them from elements of nature like the wind, and so gives them stability.

In the same way, she said, relationships among human beings can help reduce the stress of daily life and prevent heart disease. Research backs up this idea. The more healthy and cohesive the family and community, the less heart disease. I don't think anyone would disagree that we need more love in our society, but how do we get it?

I'm lacking in this area—have a hard time being dependent on people. I was always taught to do things myself. Okay, so I feel bummed out because I'm deficient. How do I start to change? What's the point in learning this stuff if it's just going to make me feel bad? I'm trying to help Dad, but will he listen, or understand, or make any changes? If I can't make changes, how can he?

She says it's okay to be driven by your work as long you like what you do. If you work too hard, however, or if you feel trapped in a job you don't like, it's bad for the heart. That makes sense to me. She said that even if I find work that I really like, it's still important to save time for close relationships, recreation, and quiet time.

All three—Dr. Frank, Dr. James, and Dr. Judy—said that being keyed up stresses the whole body and can eventually cause heart damage. Dr. Judy talked about "being in touch with your soul or with wholeness." I don't know quite what she meant.

Doctor's Notepad

Alice begins to understand why CPBP is so pervasive in Western society and to learn how people can best protect their health. The explosion of information technology and the extremely competitive nature of business today contribute to the accelerated pace of life. People expect to move more quickly and to complete projects in less time. Unrealistic expectations create a widespread sense of pressure. This time urgency encourages persistent frenetic activity and racing thoughts. Chronic over-arousal can exhaust the individual and interfere with the development and maintenance of relationships and support systems. When we feel rushed and tired we are more reactive and prone to anger.

Three different types of time disorders have been identified. They have been termed time pressure, time urgency, and hurry sickness (Allan and Scheidt, 1996; Friedman and Rosenman, 1974).

Time pressure involves the belief that one does not have enough time to do all the things they feel the need to do. This can cause feelings of anxiety and tension.

Time urgency involves the combination of time pressure with the belief that if one just goes faster they will have a better chance of getting everything done. A person starts walking, talking, eating, etc. faster and doing multiple tasks simultaneously, which can all create a tendency to be impatient and intolerant of waiting and others who move more slowly (which is most everyone). Time urgency can become a habit, and feeling a need to hurry becomes present even when there is not any time pressure.

Chronic time urgency is termed "hurry sickness." In this case, a person loses all interest in anything other than the achievement of their goals. Life becomes about quantity, rather than quality. The ability to concentrate becomes disrupted by rapid, racing thoughts; this can interfere with sleep, also. Lastly, people with hurry sickness are focused on planning for the future or handling crises or problems in the present moment; obviously, this can severely diminish their quality of life.

When a person feels good about the work she does, a busy schedule can be energizing in a positive way. Individuals and communities are healthier when they are productive. A strenuous schedule is most likely to be a health risk when a person does not like what he does, has little control of his environment or schedule, and feels trapped in the situation.

Many people overwork out of fear of the unknown, trying to create a feeling of inner security through financial security. This approach is likely to be stressful for their hearts. Most people with CPBP are driven by insecurity and anxiety. Becoming more aware of these problems can help you make healthier and more conscious decisions about your work. Do your very best to find work that you enjoy!

Sometimes people keep themselves busy as a distraction from the lack of inner peace they experience. A life of constant activity can gnaw at your spiritual sense of self. We would benefit significantly as a culture if we valued the pursuit of an integrated wholeness within each other and ourselves, instead of some external form of success.

We don't have very clear definitions or ways of measuring a person's level of wholeness. By the term "wholeness" I mean one's complete, integrated self—the true nature of the individual that includes the way she thinks and behaves. We don't have a clear definition or way of measuring a person's level of wholeness, but we do know that when little attention is paid to the soul or the person's full self in the culture at large, this lack manifests itself in fragmented relationships and communities.

We need quiet time to go inward and listen—not to the incessant chatter of the mind, but to the quiet, warm hum inside of each of us. When we are in constant motion we become a society of "human doings" and we are prone to forget how to connect with the deeper aspects of ourselves and each other.

Today's society includes complex, competitive global markets, technologically advanced communication and information systems, and increasing economic divisions—all in an atmosphere lacking in support networks. Significant numbers of people feel isolated. These trends all contribute to the current epidemic of coronary heart disease.

If you suffer from time urgency, here are some practical steps you can take:

1. Re-evaluate. Try and be aware that you have time urgency and ask yourself if your current list of things to do is worth having a heart attack over.

2. Take three deep belly breaths anytime you feel rushed (more in Chapter Five).

3. Make "to do" lists each day and rank the items in order of their priority. Things that need to be done today get an "A" ranking. The next important items get a "B." "C" means that the item can easily be put off until another day.

4. Use self-talk to reassure yourself: "I can do this" or "Its okay, the world isn't going to come to an end if I don't do everything perfectly."

5. Try to keep a realistic perspective on what you can accomplish in a given amount of time.

6. If you find it impossible to relax, you may be suffering with an anxiety disorder or some other kind of medical imbalance. In this case, please have your self evaluated by a medical professional.

7. Take time to be calm and quiet, and then take an honest look at how you are living your life. Are you living in a way that you find fulfilling and meaningful? Do you take time to develop close relationships? Do you feel a sense of connectedness within your community? Do you cultivate and tend to your spiritual life? All of these activities will improve the health of your heart.

Chapter Five

The Stress Management Coach: Coping Strategies for Optimal Health

"To bring about peace, our hearts must be at peace. Mindfulness is the practice of stopping and becoming aware of what we are thinking and doing. The more we are mindful of our thoughts, speech, and actions, the more we develop concentration. With concentration, insight into the nature of our own suffering and the suffering of others arises. We then know what to do and what not to do to live joyfully and in peace."

—Thich Nhat Hanh

"He enjoys true leisure who has time to improve his soul's estate."

—Henry David Thoreau

"Meditation heals evil thoughts, sadness, and woes."

—Hippocrates, in 400 BC

April 13, 7:30 A.M.

It's a new day, and I'll make sure to see Dad. I must also try to return the calls from my friends. I should try Dr. Judy's suggestions for preventing heart disease, because I don't want to have my heart give out on me in the middle of my life and go through what Dad is going through!

I feel selfish being worried about me while Dad is recuperating, but I like what Dr. Judy said yesterday about inner peace. It's frustrating to learn which feelings increase my chances of developing heart disease and to acknowledge that I suffer from a lack of inner peace, mood swings, and a tendency to get angry and to isolate myself, and not know what the solutions are. Okay, so I don't have inner peace. How many people do? I can feel myself starting to get mad. I'd rather not know this stuff.

It's time to see Dad.

April 13, 3:00 P.M.

Dad looked so tired today, it really upset me. I went to see him, thinking that he was going home soon. He surprised me by talking a little about how he felt. I wish I'd known what to say. He admitted that he feels disoriented and out-of-sorts. One minute he was fine, and, in the blink of an eye, he found himself in the hospital having open-heart surgery. He feels tired, and he's bothered because he has ugly scars.

They scare me. He has scars on his chest from where they opened him up, and one down his leg where they took out an artery to use in his heart. They make the hair on the back of my neck stand up. I was glad he talked to me, but I felt helpless and lost. I don't know whether my research project will help him or not.

The doctor who teaches stress management in the cardiac rehab program at the hospital came in and introduced himself. He wanted to tell Dad about his program, but Dad was belligerent. He wouldn't listen, and was irritated that I encouraged the guy to keep on talking. Because

Dad was getting so agitated, the doctor and I agreed to meet in his office for a short time tomorrow.

April 14, 4:00 P.M.

Great meeting today. The doctor had a calm appealing way about him, and he did give me some advice about stress management. He recommended relaxation, meditation, breathing exercises, physical exercises, and a low-stress diet.

Unfortunately, when I asked him what he meant by a low-stress diet he said that I should consult a nutritionist about my own eating plan, because each person has individual needs. Generally, however, he recommended the usual: lots of fresh vegetables, fruits, whole grains, beans, legumes, and nuts. He said to keep animal products and processed vegetable oils to a minimum. I think I can do this.

Like the other experts, he said that the standard risk factors of smoking, eating too much, overusing alcohol, and having high blood pressure are really symptoms of stress. His overall prescription for preventing and recovering from heart disease is to have a positive, realistic outlook. He said that living the way he suggests is medicine that people can take daily without any negative consequences.

When I asked him how he gets people to make these changes, he said that he doesn't. People have to want to change. One of the reasons he likes working with cardiac patients is that many of them are so frightened that they are open to making changes. He said people can change their lifestyles and attitudes superficially by making changes in their diets, exercising, not smoking, etc., but that unless they look deeper inside themselves to uncover what is fueling their destructive habits the changes won't benefit them fully.

He used the example of a perfectionist. Because the details of life can never be completely controlled or made perfect, the need to make everything perfect can create a lot of anxiety and stress. Even if I practiced his stress-reduction exercises daily, I would return to trying to control every little thing in my life; this would be superficial stress reduction. He said I need to understand why I approach things the way I do and change that method.

I admitted to him that I get angry when things don't go my way and asked him to show me how to change this. I gave him some examples. I get mad at rude drivers and upset at having to wait in a line.

He said I can choose to see things differently. When a driver cuts in front of me and scares me half to death, instead of having a hostile reaction I can choose to respond with acceptance and compassion. I can give the person the benefit of the doubt. Maybe the guy just got news that a family member was in a terrible accident, or maybe he'll be fired if he doesn't get to work on time.

He said I should assume that people have a reason for the things they do, and I should not judge them. It's bad for my health to get mad, and anger doesn't help the situation anyway. I need to turn my feelings around and wish the bad drivers a safe journey.

The average person living in an urban area, he told me, has about thirty unexpected stressors a day! Imagine if you have the habit of getting angry every time one happens. If you're trying to calm your system and one of these stressors happens, you can use the opportunity to practice calmness and understanding. You can choose to have a peaceful perspective.

I had an opportunity to try this on the way home, and it did work— to some extent. I was able to calm down, but it was hard work. If I really commit myself and practice regularly, though, I guess it'll become a habit, just as getting angry is a habit now. Finally, I am starting to understand that I have to learn to regulate myself so that I don't get sick or too aggravated.

Staying healthy shouldn't be so much work, but I guess I might be happier, too, if I didn't get mad so often. My heart would feel better if I lived the way he described. Sometimes, though, when I get quiet and calm I feel my heart hurting, and I'd rather stay busy and irritated, because it kind of numbs me from my own pain.

He said emotional tension builds in the body even without our knowing it. Sometimes people get angry easily because unconsciously they hurt about something they haven't dealt with. They may not even know they're upset, but these feelings come up when something else happens. When I realize that I'm feeling tense, I'm supposed to pay attention to what I'm thinking and feeling—what my attitude is about what's happening right then.

He gave me some tips on breathing exercises and meditation. He likes to keep it all as simple as possible. He said that whatever I focus my mind on will become part of me, so if I practice calming exercises, even when I'm out and about in the world, I can cultivate a better attitude in general.

In the car, at a red light, I am to turn off the radio and breathe in and out deeply and slowly several times before the light changes. I should pause briefly between inhaling and exhaling and notice how quiet the transition is.

Before making a telephone call or beginning a conversation with someone I should breathe in and out deeply and slowly three times. As I write this, I'm aware of how shallow my breathing is. He said that cardiac patients usually have shallow breathing styles. I took a couple of slow, deep breaths and felt as if I was stretching my chest and lungs. How shallowly I must be breathing most of the time! After another couple of these deep breaths I do feel calmer and a little energized. Maybe there's something to this. I just have to remember to do it.

I asked him what happens when I become more aware of what I'm feeling because I do his calming exercises. What am I supposed to do with painful emotions? He had a good answer: the emotions don't go away, but I can learn to cope with them in a healthy way. Deep, slow breathing and meditation that help calm and clear the mind can release emotional and physical tension so I can deal more effectively with the thoughts that upset me.

Emotions need to be released, and if I do this in a healthy way they lose intensity. More importantly, I'm supposed to accept the feelings, breathe through them, listen to myself, and learn to understand myself better.

I asked him, "What if I just can't do this? What if I can't relax, no matter how hard I try?" Once again he had a good answer. Vigorous physical exercise releases endorphins that create a feeling of calm and well-being. Active meditation exercises like yoga, tai chi, qi gong, and Pilates all combine body movement, breathing, and mental stillness. I just don't know how I'd find the time to do these, but I can start to work on my attitude, and that's the most important change.

He said that developing a positive outlook and reducing what he calls "the typical CPBP cynical, antagonistic and gloomy outlook on life, which promotes emotional isolation and alienation from other people" are most important, because anger or happiness come from our perceptions of how we should feel.

I surprised myself by being honest with him, and complained that if I could have done these things, I would have. He admitted that change takes effort and practice, but said it's easier to implement change than live a miserable life. I wouldn't say I'm miserable, at least not all the time. Sure, I'm a little worried and stressed and sometimes border on miserable, especially if things aren't going the way I want them to.

April 14, 9:30 P.M.

I just came home from visiting Dad. He still looked tired, and I still didn't know what to say, so I didn't say anything. I felt inspired by my meeting with the stress management coach, but I didn't know how to tell Dad about it. I started to wonder if all the information I'm gathering is really any help, or just another distraction? Maybe I should try using what the coach taught me today. At least I can see whether it can help, and if it does work I can suggest it to Dad. I'll try taking those three deep breaths.

April 14, 10:00 P.M.

The three breaths did help a little, but then Mrs. Orangey called, wanting to know if I needed her help to get Dad home two days from now. Kind, but I told her no. I did ask her to visit him tomorrow if she could, because I have to catch up at work and meet a psychoneuroimmunologist. What a name! Still, he was great on the phone—enthusiastic about preventing heart disease. Instead of making me feel dumb because I don't know what he does, he said he'll explain it to me.

Anyway, the breathing technique did help. I was probably nicer to Mrs. Orangey than I sometimes am. I feel better about myself when I'm calmer.

All I did was to sit back in my favorite chair and breathe in and out, slowly and deeply, focusing my mind on my breathing and noticing the pause between the inhaling and the exhaling. It *is* quiet there. I breathed in and out three times, quieting my mind by concentrating on the breaths. At first I realized how tense I am, and then I started to relax a bit.

If I learned the practice he called "mindfulness," maybe I'd experience greater relief, but it takes too much time. I'm not trying to be a Buddha; I'm just trying to feel better—and I do feel a little less worried.

Doctor's Notepad

Alice learns practical hands-on strategies for dealing with stress that can help reduce her likelihood of developing heart disease. Mainly, there are two types of stress: external and internal. External stress is things outside of our control, e.g. long lines, traffic, weather, war, etc. Internal stress involves our perception of what we are experiencing. Our perception is influenced by our thoughts, emotions, biology, and spiritual orientation. We can adjust our way of seeing the world and our experiences to a more accepting and positive attitude; this can reduce our stress level. For example, there are many ways that we can respond to the news report that Americans can expect terrorist acts to befall upon the United States in the near future. We decide it is unsafe to leave our houses except when absolutely necessary, and we become angry and depressed. Or we can decide that it is a reminder of how precious life is and cherish each day of life that we presently have. This is an example of an attitude of gratitude and being in the present moment.

The stress management techniques presented here have to do with quieting the chatter in the mind and calming the body. We must get quiet enough inside to be able to hear our thoughts in order to increase our awareness of what we are saying to ourselves; only then can we adjust our thoughts accordingly. It is not the stressful stimuli that create illness; it is our reaction to the stimuli.

Practicing stress reduction exercises can reduce the standard risk factors and help extend and improve the duration and quality of our lives. Scientific research has shown that quieting the mind is associated with wellness.

Practicing acceptance of our feelings and cultivating a positive attitude will help. Below you will find some exercises to help calm the mind and body and begin to retrain yourself to handle stress differently

Some exercises for stress reduction, relaxation, and inner peace:

1. Basic breath:	Take three slow, deep breaths any time you think of it.
2. Belly breathing:	Put one hand on your chest and one hand on your lower belly. Take a deep breath and see which moves more, your chest or your belly. When we are stressed, anxious or tired, we tend to breathe shallowly from the chest. Breathing into your lower belly brings more oxygen into the body. Practice deep breathing with your lower belly moving with your breath more dramatically than your chest. Do this for 60 seconds to 5 minutes and you will notice that you feel calmer and more relaxed.
3. Count and breathe:	Breathe in through your nose, count "one," and then breathe out through your mouth and say "and." Do this at least ten times.
4. Ahhh:	Breathe in and out, deeply and slowly, and say and hold the word "ahhhh". Do this for five minutes. Practice this out loud and simultaneously with people you love for optimal healing benefits.
5. Notice the air:	Breathe in deeply through your nostrils and exhale slowly through your nostrils. Notice the feeling of the air as it moves through your nostrils. Notice how the air is cooler on the inhale and warmer on the exhale. Quiet your mind and focus your

attention on the temperature as it moves in and out of your nostrils for 1-5 minutes.

6. Little friend: When you are sitting, breathing, and quieting your mind, sometimes you may notice that you feel angry, sad, and other things. You may also notice negative thoughts. Accept your feelings and thoughts and breathe into them. Try saying hello to them, "Hello, my little friends." Try to understand your emotion or thought without judging. Be kind toward your yourself. Once you are aware of how you feel or think, accept it and then let it go—just like you might watch a cloud in the sky go by. You don't usually follow it or try jumping on and going for a ride. Let your thoughts and emotions go; don't grasp onto them and make them who you are. Most thoughts and emotions are temporary. If you accept them and then let go, your emotions and thoughts are less likely to make you sick. You may also feel more peaceful.

7. Rhythmic breathing: Sit in a comfortable position with your back straight and your eyes lightly closed. Focus your attention on your breathing—the inhalation, exhalation, and the shifting in between. Practice this breathing for five minutes each day. Follow the natural cycle of your breathing without judging the pattern of depth

or respiration. Continue to notice the rhythm of the cycle. This basic method of relaxation can help to harmonize your body, mind, and spirit.

8. Single focus:

Choose a soothing word, sound, or image, and sit quietly, focusing your mind on it. When other thoughts come into your mind, let them move on by like a bus; don't jump on and go for the ride. Keep bringing your attention back to the word, sound, or image. Focusing the mind on nature can be restful and restorative. Picture a beautiful place, a flower, or the sky brightening at sunrise. Listen to the song of a bird, the rhythm of the ocean, or the sound of a fountain. If you are religious, you can focus on a religious symbol or a favorite prayer.

9. Guided Imagery:

Stop everything and be quiet. Go to a place where you are resting, but not sleeping. Settle into the relaxation, letting your body soften. Let your chest soften. Bring your awareness to the feeling in your body and in your chest area. Breathe. Bring your awareness to the blood vessels as they pump a vital blood supply to your heart organ—and take in a deep breath. Bring fresh oxygen into your expanding lungs and into your blood stream, supplying oxygenated blood to your heart and body. See the blood circulating, pumping smoothly, through your cardiovascular system.

Take a deep breath and become aware of the subtle relaxation that comes with your deep breathing. Breathe in slowly and deeply into your lower belly, exhaling slowly, pushing all of the air temporarily out of your belly and your lungs. Empty yourself out. With each breath, think about oxygenating your cells—every cell in your body—feeding your body, soothing your body, energizing your spirit with each breath. As you exhale, focus on letting go of anything that you are holding on to, letting go and experience the peace and stillness of the present moment.

Any time you notice your mind start to wander off, bring your focus back to the breath, to softening the body, and being in the peace and stillness of the present moment. Continue practicing slow, natural, deep breaths, letting go of anything bothering you or any concerns you may have; focus on your breathing, relaxing, keeping your awareness on just this: in this brief, present, eternal, moment, practicing for 5 minutes or more. Every time you notice that your thoughts are off wandering, gently bring your awareness back to your breath, breathing the life force into your body.

Make a commitment to practice one of these exercises as a way of improving your well-being, rather than just one more thing added to your list of chores. Become more aware of what you are thinking, feeling, and believing. This can be very beneficial to your relationship with yourself and your loved ones and to your overall quality of life.

Chapter Six

The Psychoneuroimmunologist: How the Mind, Brain, and Body Communicate

"The perception of love itself…may turn out to be a core bio-psychosocial-spiritual buffer, reducing the negative impact of stressors and pathogens and promoting immune function and healing."

—Harvard researchers Dr. Stanley King, Dr.s Russek, and Dr. Gary Schwartz

April 15, 8:00 P.M.

I actually feel like I am making some progress. It was fascinating meeting with Psychoneuroimmunologist Dr. Gene. He helped me put together what everyone's been talking about.

He said, "Psychoneuroimmunology is the study of interactions between the brain and the immune system." Our thoughts affect the whole body, including the cardiovascular system. He amazed me by saying that there's no difference between "mind" and "body." They are different words for energy.

Everything, including our body, is made up of energy. The mind/body is one energy system with zillions of atoms all talking to each other. Negative thoughts are negative messages sent through this whole system. Our mind influences our neurochemicals, hormones, immune system, and everything else in the body. Lack of love can make our hearts sick.

If I want to stay healthy, I have to be aware of what I'm thinking all the time, and I don't know if I can or want to do that.

April 15, 8:30 P.M.

I was interrupted by a phone call from Dad's acquaintance Sam Jones, who wanted to know how he's doing. Mr. Jones wasn't sure if he should bother Dad at the hospital or not. I told him Dad's going home tomorrow and I'm sure Dad would be glad to hear from him. I felt sad for Mr. Jones. I happen to know that he's a very lonely guy. Since his wife died, he hardly ever talks to anyone. Maybe he's shy. I know Dad likes him.

I think I'm making progress because I started to feel a little irritated when the phone rang and then a little more irritated when he asked me such a silly question (of course Dad would want to hear from him), but I became aware of the irritation right away and stopped it. Mr. Jones is lonely and he was just trying to be kind. I feel sympathetic toward him, which is a lot better than being angry.

Dr. Gene took me through a good exercise. He asked me to think of something that I'm worried about. Of course I picked Dad. The doctor asked me to relax, so I did a couple of minutes of a breathing exercise. First he asked me to imagine my dad never feeling better again, never again being quite himself. I did, and I felt so sad I wanted to cry. Second, he told me to close my eyes and imagine my dad completely recovered, better than ever. I felt happy and noticed a physical change in my body.

Then I was supposed to imagine my father and me being angry at each other. I couldn't imagine my being angry at Dad right now, but I did imagine him mad at me, and I felt a wall going up around myself, like my heart was hurting. The doctor said, "Now imagine you know that no matter what happens, even if your Dad gets upset with you, he loves you and is committed to the relationship, and the two of you will always work things out." When I imagined that I felt love, calm, contentment, and warmth in my heart.

So people are energy, and when we are connected to each other our energy is connected. He believes that I can help Dad by thinking good thoughts about him or praying for him. Cardiologists did a study that showed that patients recover more quickly when people pray for them. I'd like to believe that's true, but it also suggests I have a big responsibility toward other people. When I feel negative toward other people I might create more stress in the world, with negative energy fueling negative energy.

April 16, 6:30 A.M.

I got up early. I sat outside on my porch, reviewing my notes from all the interviews so far. I did a couple minutes of relaxation—breathing, quieting my mind, focusing on my breathing. It's funny how something that feels good is still hard to do for very long.

I'm taking Dad home today. I will go over to his house first, put flowers around, clean things up, and get food in the house. I'm sure he'll be glad to be home.

April 16, 3:00 P.M.

I sat in my car outside of the pharmacy, shook up. After waiting in line for an infuriating fifteen minutes to pick up Dad's prescriptions, they still weren't ready. They were supposed to be ready this morning, and I allowed extra time because the pharmacy is always so slow. Then, when they didn't have Dad's prescriptions they didn't even apologize. I started to blow up, but then I got frightened at how mad I was and realized that it wasn't going to help. I wanted to scream at them, "Get me those medicines now!" but I knew they wouldn't move any faster, no matter how much I tried to bully them.

I just about blew a gasket when they said the prescriptions would be ready in about thirty minutes. Who has thirty minutes to sit around waiting for prescriptions? What are they thinking?

I marched out to my car, and here I am, scribbling on my notepad when I should be practicing breathing or meditating, but it does help just to write about a problem, and now I can take deep breaths. I must admit that a month ago I might have been even angrier with them. I'm sure they saw that I wasn't happy, and the other people in line smiled at me sympathetically. They understood. That helped a little bit. We are all in the same boat.

April 16, 9:00 P.M.

Dad is all settled in and seems glad to be home. I made him dinner and we had a nice time. He told me about his cardiac rehab class and that he now knows about the standard risk factors to watch out for, including stress and social isolation. I asked him what he had learned about stress. He said that it's bad, and we both cracked up! Seems like a long time since we had done that.

He said that at first he was irritated with the cardiac support group because they all had to introduce themselves and talk about their lives without talking about their work. This was tough for him, since work is his main focus in life, but he was surprised that he enjoyed hearing about the other people, and he even liked some of them. Since the leader of the group promised that attending the group would help prevent another heart attack, Dad agreed to continue to go to it.

He's worried, though, about losing his edge. His attitude works for him in the business world, and he's afraid that he won't be as successful without it. I encouraged him by joking that even if he gave up half of his edge he'd still be a tiger. He seemed to appreciate my trying to pump him up, but I don't think he bought it.

I explained that I'm trying to have a more positive attitude, and it's not as easy as it sounds. He nodded, and I felt less alone, as if he really understood. I said something else about being positive, and he chuckled and rolled his eyes. Before I'd have felt hurt, but now I was able to smile. He seemed to realize that he was chuckling at something I meant seriously, and stopped. He even asked me some earnest questions about my research, told me that he'd like to see me more often, and hugged me first when I said good-bye.

Tears come to my eyes as I am writing. I almost lost the chance to really know Dad. Because he is home now and was warm to me tonight, I feel as if we might really become closer. I didn't realize how important he is to me, but I guess the prospect of losing him made me realize how much he means to me. Maybe something good will come out of all of this. It will if Dad takes better care of himself and I learn to calm down and take time to open my heart to the people I love.

The Psychoneuroimmunologist: How the Mind, Brain, and Body Communicate

Doctor's Notepad

Psychoneuroimmunology is the study of how the mind and the body communicate. The mind and body function together, united by messenger molecules that are the communication channels of the human system. These messenger molecules relay information back and forth among our thoughts, emotions, and cells, ultimately even influencing our genetic structure.

Messenger molecules—or neurotransmitters—are chemicals created by our brain cells. Thoughts are specific energy or brain-wave patterns that stimulate chemical production in the brain. Each thought we have generates synchronized neural oscillations that release specific chemicals in the brain and body. Synchronized neural oscillations are the simultaneous electrical charges among neurons that translate into chemical secretions and then transform the energy experience in the body.

These chemicals—or messenger molecules—communicate between neurons, and then between our neurons and nerves. These communications affect the whole nervous system, and thus affect the cardiovascular system.

We are just beginning to understand how our mind and body function as one entity. Our thoughts affect the biochemistry of our whole system. The human body, mind, and spirit form one interconnected system.

A negative communication translates to a physical negation of the life force in the body, in contrast to a positive communication that ends up stimulating and encouraging the life force. Since the cells in our body are constantly replacing themselves, our mental perspective affects the energy of our constantly reorganizing, regenerating body. Repetitive thought patterns and behavior tendencies can accumulate over time to affect the body positively or destructively.

For example, consider the fight-or-flight reaction I mentioned earlier. It was very effective many thousands of years ago when we had to be on the alert for dangerous predators. Some psychologists think of the cortex and sub-cortex as the new brain and the old brain respectively, and speculate that evolution has produced a whole population of human beings who continue to operate with the old brain, because those with well-developed old brains would have survived and been able to reproduce over the years. In today's stressful urban world, the same survival mechanism (fight-or-flight) that used to be adaptive can become a suicidal overdose on adrenaline and pessimism.

The time has come for the brain to adapt to a different world. We now need to wire optimism into our regular behaviors in daily living. The time is now for the win-win philosophy to become a style of living for human beings.

The following study speaks to the power of consciousness and the connection all human beings have to one another. A cardiologist took two groups of acute cardiac patients and gave them identical, top-notch medical care. The first names and descriptions of each patient in one of the groups were given to various prayer groups. The members were asked to pray for these people, but were not told why they were praying for them. Those in the group of patients who were being prayed for recovered at a significantly faster rate than those in the other patient group.

The world of technology has learned miraculous methods of channeling energy, for example, in the burgeoning field of wireless technology. We human beings can learn to use our own energy effectively for our own health and well-being and that of our loved ones. Some of the most powerful ways to take care of your energy for optimal health and relationships are: learn to practice compassion and forgiveness; develop a positive, healthy belief in yourself; and appreciate the gift of life on a daily basis.

One definition of compassion is "the giving of understanding and unconditional acceptance with a desire to alleviate suffering." When you feel angry with someone or yourself, try to feel compassion for that person instead. You may not be able to do this right away; sometimes we have to let ourselves be angry, but as soon as you can feel compassion, do that. It will help you heal. Your cardiovascular system will soften and relax and your blood will flow more smoothly through your veins. When you experience anger, it is also important to accept that feeling and take care of yourself. Be careful not to become angry with yourself for being angry (this can be vicious cycle). If you are gentle with yourself and return to compassion as soon as possible, your health and relationships will be better.

Remember that according to physicists everything is energy. Try not to harbor anger or resentments. Try to be understanding of other people and their pain or weaknesses and be forgiving. By doing this you will be taking good care of your own energy.

Discover what your own internal conflicts may be and try to resolve them. Counseling can help uncover existing inner conflicts and to solve problems. Regular relaxation or meditation can help keep your energy balanced. Mental calm and feelings of well-being translate to the cells of the body in a way that promotes wellness. Also, spending time with yourself, taking time to listen to your individual inner world, can help release feelings and thoughts that are causing stress.

Allow your self to give and receive healthy love.

Chapter Seven

The Psychologist: Behavioral Medicine

"When people begin to be real with their feelings, things happen in their bodies' physiology that encourage healing."

—Harvey Zarren, M.D., board certified cardiologist and associate clinical professor of medicine at Tufts University School of Medicine

April 17, 6:30 A.M.

I feel energized this morning, relieved to have Dad home. I'll take a few minutes to be quiet and read the paper, go to work, and then go out to dinner with Jill. I feel guilty that I've not been tending to our friendship, but I don't even want to meet her tonight. I'd rather stay late at work and make up for lost time—or visit Dad. I'll definitely check in with him by phone and hope that he'll have a visitor, then offer to bring him dinner on my way to see Jill. I just don't want to have to deal with it if Jill's mad at me.

Maybe I should stop drinking coffee. One cup and I'm buzzing, already worrying about the coming day and I feel like crawling back into bed and pulling the covers over my head.

Okay, I'll try one of the breathing techniques that the stress doc taught me. I guess I can spare five minutes from my morning. It's hard to sit and do nothing with everything I have to do and not enough time or energy to do it, but I guess that's always the case with me. I'll sit in the corner of my little couch and spend five to ten minutes just focusing on breathing in and out, trying to let my mind go blank.

April 17, 7:15 A.M.

That felt really good! I'll try to remember to do my breathing for five minutes before I meet Jill. I'm also going to stop by the bookstore for the books the stress doctor recommended. Maybe I'll get copies for Dad, too.

I have an appointment with a psychologist tomorrow to discuss CPBP. She calls herself a "cardiac psychologist," specializing in working with heart patients and teaching them how to live in a way to prevent heart disease. I wonder if she'll have anything new to add to my growing understanding.

April 17, 10:30 P.M.

It was a productive day. Mrs. Orangey brought dinner over to Dad and kept him company. Tomorrow I'll do it.

I had a good time with Jill. She wasn't mad at me and thought I was silly to think she was, and said I had every reason to be preoccupied with Dad. I told her about interviewing the different doctors. She thought that was a great idea.

Jill and I met in high school, so she knows me pretty well. When I told her what I was learning, she laughed and said that I could really benefit from practicing this stuff. I felt defensive, but she's right.

After an hour and a half I started to get nervous, thinking about everything that I need to do at home to get ready for tomorrow's meeting, but instead of getting restless and cranky like I usually do, I watched what was happening inside me and remembered to take good breaths. This helped bring me back to the moment with Jill. I didn't try to fight off my thoughts about needing to be doing something else; I just noticed them and they eased up.

Usually she can tell when I'm getting restless and she says, "Well, I can see I've lost you. I must've rattled on too long." I always feel badly when she says that, because she's so good at listening to me. She didn't seem to notice that I was focusing on my breathing, and I was able to listen to her while I was doing it. It feels good to be applying what I'm learning. I hate that feeling of getting tense when I'm with family or friends. These things that I'm learning may help me be a better person—more patient and available to those I care about as an added benefit.

April 18, 12:00 P.M.

I'm sitting in the reception area, waiting for the psychologist. Why do I feel anxious about talking with her? Am I afraid that she'll be able to read my mind and see how selfish I've become? I started this project for Dad, but now I'm doing it for me. I shouldn't care what she thinks. Oh, boy, I'm really nervous! I will spend a few minutes being quiet and breathing. That should help.

April 18, 3:00 P.M.

I liked Dr. Rose, the shrink. Her message was essentially the same as the others', but she described the high-risk person in more depth. People with CPBP have a strong need for achievement and put a lot of pressure on themselves. She said that deep down they don't feel very good about themselves. They feel they have to prove their worth. She said that hostility is one of the most important risk factors. Angry people are likely to be lonely because the anger affects their relationships. People with CPBP see emotions as getting in the way of doing what they want to do.

Dr. Rose thinks that anger is a quick cover-up of other emotions. It's easier to get angry than to feel sadness, fear, or hurt. This is something for me to think about. She said people with CPBP don't know what to do with their feelings, so they just push them away, and then the body responds negatively. People with CPBP mistrust other people.

April 18, 9:00 P.M.

Dr. Rose tied together what everyone else has talked about. Being self-aware is really important, but she called it "self-intimacy." I like that. It's a relief to live only one moment at a time. Bringing my awareness into the "now moment" helps me really experience the present, and I can handle whatever I'm feeling if I focus on the here and now, instead of overwhelming myself with thoughts and worries about the past or the future. Life feels fuller and richer when I'm tuned in to it one moment at a time. I think she called it "mindfulness." Taking a few deep breaths helps me do this.

She taught me about the power of the imagination. I didn't think that I had a good imagination, but she told me if I can worry, I can imagine. Worrying is imagining or fantasizing. She's right. I spin these stories of terrible things that could happen, and then I feel upset by the possibilities; then I look for things that will prove my negative expectations.

Dr. Rose suggested I imagine what I want to happen and feel as if it has already happened—programming myself for the positive. I am supposed to look for cues in my environment that will help create a positive outcome. It makes good sense to me, but why isn't it easier to do?

She said changing the emotional programs we have set up inside ourselves takes time and effort. If we pretend not to let things bother us, as we always did in my family, these feelings we don't own build up inside us.

How do I go from being numb to everything except my anger to feeling my other feelings, and from being stressed out to being calm? She said that first I have to be aware of what I'm feeling. Some people are so good at ignoring how they feel that they end up with migraines or exhaustion at the end of the day and don't know why.

I asked her about me. What can I do when I'm driving, a car darts in front of me, and I get mad? She said I need to accept my response as normal and try to forgive myself and the inconsiderate driver.

To relieve tough feelings I can talk with a supportive friend, write about them, or exercise. She suggested vigorous physical exercise five times a week—regular stretching or yoga, progressive muscle relaxation, breathing exercises, meditation, massage, and acupuncture—as ways of decreasing stress.

At least massage and acupuncture are new ideas. I got the name of an acupuncturist who specializes in anxiety, stress, and heart problems. The psychologist confirmed what I had already heard—that changing the way I think can decrease stress—but she did tell me to look at the facts. That sounds more sensible than all this fantasy-making.

April 19, 7:30 A.M.

I feel a little overwhelmed this morning. I need to get to work and make stuff happen, look in on Dad, stay in touch with my friends whom I've been neglecting, pay my bills, and on and on. I've added breathing techniques and meditation to the list. Ideally I should do regular exercises, and work on my self-awareness. I can't believe how lazy I am. I'm finally getting some answers, and I won't even use them. That's pathetic.

The psychologist said I need to start hearing what I say to myself privately, and if the thoughts are negative I must stop myself and replace them with positive ones. I'm beginning to hear the mean things I say to myself about myself—like a constant whisper in my head.

She suggested that when I think, Ugh, I have to go to work. I'm so behind I'll never catch up. They're probably mad at me, to say to myself instead, "I can do this," over and over. I can see how I can change my attitude over time if I really work on it. She promised it would help free up my energy so I'd feel less weighed down and be able to do my work better.

Also, she said I should look inside myself to see if I have some deep beliefs about my self-image, my self-doubt, and lack of confidence, and perhaps talk with a professional counselor to see if my negative view of myself is realistic or not.

I closed my eyes when she told me to, and imagined how it would feel if I believed in myself. I felt energized, strong, and excited about doing the things I want to do. She recommended that I practice that feeling in my imagination as if it's already true.

I'd feel better if I took the mental energy that I use to worry and imagined positive outcomes instead, she says. She calls worrying "negative imagination."

She gave me the example of a man who worries about money. He imagines his wife is worried about money, too, but she's not. She really wants more quality time with him. By the end of the day he's in a bad mood and not sure why. The guy needs to communicate with his wife, and if he says nicer things to himself like "I am lovable" and "I'm a good husband," he's going to be in a better mood and will be more loving when he gets home. She says that if he stops the negative chatter in his mind and makes his thinking more neutral he won't be as worn out at the end of the day.

I asked her how a distrustful and angry person can change. I'm always expecting people to leave me. She said that we develop belief systems about which we are and what the world is like, and then we see everything that happens through these filters. These belief systems are developed in childhood, created by the way a kid interprets experiences.

She said I can change this if I want to; I just have to be aware of my beliefs. It sounds too easy.

April 19, 12:00 P.M.

It's lunch break. Jill called and wants to get together. I told her I've just got too much work to catch up on. She told me that I need a break. I know she's trying to be supportive, but I feel pressured. How does she know what I need?

The morning was productive, so I feel better. I've been thinking about my meeting with the psychologist. I was an emotional kid, but in my family, part of being a good kid was to keep quiet and not be any trouble. No one liked dealing with strong emotions, so I learned to keep them to myself. That's what everyone else seemed to do, too. I got strokes for good grades and being independent.

Now I realize I don't let anyone get close to me, and I don't even know myself because I try to ignore what I'm feeling and I just push through it. I want to accomplish so many things, and it seems self-indulgent to pay attention to my inner self. Getting a manicure seems more acceptable than meditating.

It's hard for me to sit still and meditate. My mind runs all over the place. Maybe part of me thinks in some warped way that it's too self-indulgent to meditate, even though I know meditation will help. I believe what these doctors are all saying, but no one else has ever said anything like this, so I always feel like I should be doing something else. I worry too much about what other people think of me. I've never had a relationship where I felt loved and accepted just for myself. My fantasy is that love should be a kind of grace within and between people, as natural and flowing as the relationship between the moon and the ocean tides. Is this just romantic nonsense?

April 20, 7:00 A.M.

I visited Dad last night. He was cranky and distant. I worried that I'd done something wrong, but I knew I hadn't. I could spend more time with him, but I never know how he's going to feel or act, so I guess I avoid him and then feel bad about it. I can't win, no matter what. He's always been moody, now that I think about it, and I take his moods personally.

I will try one of Dr. Susan's ideas for me. My notes say to make a positive, present tense statement about how I want to feel so I can reprogram myself. Okay, "I am lovable, even if Dad doesn't always treat me like I am. I am lovable!"

That feels nice. I did it. I said it over and over to myself and took slow, deep breaths and felt my stomach relax and calmness spread inside my body. I felt peaceful. It is good way to start the day.

April 24, 9:00 P.M.

I haven't written for a few days. Dad's doing better. He acts as if nothing happened. It's frustrating. I know he still isn't himself, but he gets mad when I ask him how he is. I want to talk with him about our relationship and make it better, but he won't let me. I'm anxious and angry.

I tried to sit quietly and breathe through my feelings, trying to experience them, accept how I feel, and let go of the pain as I exhale. Dr. Rose's prescription helped ease the tension. Dad is who he is, and I can't change him, though it hurts my heart to realize that I'll probably never have the kind of relationship I'd like to have with him. Accepting my own feelings and being close with my self while I'm having these feelings does feel better. I feel less lonely and desperate. Maybe this is the self-intimacy Dr. Susan was talking about.

April 25, 6:30 A.M.

It is a beautiful morning. I'm sitting on the deck, practicing some deep breathing and quieting my mind by watching nature. A little yellow-breasted sparrow sitting on a nearby tree branch is looking at me. A fresh grassy scent is in the morning air, and new flowers are budding on the apricot tree. There's something healing about filling my lungs with air, slowly and deeply, resting my mind on my breath, and touching stillness for even a second.

I just had a clear feeling that Dad really does love me. Even though it's sad that he can't love me the way I want him to, it feels warm and peaceful to think that he does love me, even though he doesn't always show it.

Doctor's Notepad

Underlying the Coronary-Prone Behavior Pattern is a harsh, self-critical inner voice. People with CPBP usually have deep insecurities that are perpetuated by their tendency to whip themselves into constant activity. They find it difficult to relax and feel at peace because this inner voice never lets up on them, and all of the external achievement and material acquisition in the world will not help. This inner voice can also interfere with their ability to form intimate relationships.

People with CPBP tend to be impatient, perfectionists, and prone to hostility in situations that don't go their way. They feel the need to be successful or perfect in order to qualify for love and acceptance.

Thoughts affect our beliefs and emotions, and beliefs and emotions affect our thoughts. Negative thoughts can create negative emotions, and visa versa.

The first step is to increase your awareness of your negative thoughts. When you catch yourself having them, accept that it is there and think of a counter thought—one that is positive, rational, and cancels or balances out the negative. A counselor, therapist, or coach can be helpful with this process.

Taking a few minutes each day to spend in quiet meditation, which can be as simple as quieting the mind and focusing on breathing deeply in and out, can help cultivate more self-awareness and inner calm. Self-awareness offers the opportunity to begin making positive changes.

Acknowledging and accepting your feelings is important, because emotions are energy, and when the natural flow of energy is repeatedly obstructed because of fear or a lack of awareness, the potential for the development of disease increases.

When the human system is unobstructed, it has an amazing natural capacity for healing. For example, if you're upset about something that happened in a relationship and you hold the feeling in, it can grow even stronger. The ability to talk about your feelings and to be listened to and to be understood is healthy. Communication with the person involved can be especially helpful, depending on the situation. The intensity of the emotion actually diminishes as you release it, clearing the energy system.

People with CPBP don't know what to do with their feelings. They tend to mistrust other people, so they're reluctant to be vulnerable by exposing their emotions. Nevertheless, they can deny what they're feeling for only a limited time before the truth explodes in an outburst of anger or tears—or a heart attack.

Ideally, you want to handle your emotions in a moderate way. This requires first that you become aware of how you feel. Then, at an appropriate moment and in a calm way, you might choose to tell a caring friend about those feelings. When you share a difficult feeling with someone who really listens and cares, the intensity of the emotion naturally decreases.

Each one of us has an ongoing internal dialogue. We talk to ourselves all the time. We conjure up images, ideas, and fantasies, and imagine how we would feel if they were real. People who tend to be optimistic usually imagine positive things, while depressed pessimistic folks imagine painful, negative scenarios that might never happen. Our self-image and our world view are developed through our experiences and interpretations of events. When we vividly imagine an experience and then feel the emotions that might go along with it, this becomes part of our experience. We can, however, develop a habit of positive thinking.

Say to yourself, "I am vibrant and alive," or "I am in excellent health," or "I am calm and well." Imagine that the statement is true at this very moment. Repeat the statement to yourself as you take deep, slow breaths. You will feel more energetic.

Close, caring relationships and a supportive community are excellent preventative medicine for heart disease. People who have CPBP tend to put their work or independent activities before relationships. While they would like to have closeness with people, their lifestyle often prevents it. Actually, loving relationships don't necessarily have to interfere with a person's drive for achievement. Supportive and energizing connections can enhance success.

While there is nothing wrong with wanting to achieve and become the best one can be, it's important to recognize that we're all works in progress until the day we die. We grow and improve, then we flail about, learning, sometimes feeling as if we're slipping backwards, and then we grow some more. Being a human being is about experiencing the mystery and beauty of life and enjoying, loving, and growing as much as possible along the way. It is not about trying to become perfect in some external way.

Chapter Eight

The Acupuncturist:
The Eastern Mind/Body Approach
to Heart Health

"We now know that the heart, the blood, the mind, and the emotional state are all interdependent."

—Diana Wisdom, Ph.D., cardiac psychologist

"A mental disturbance provoking pain, excessive joy, hope, or anxiety extends to the heart, where it affects temper and rate."

—William Harvey, 1628,
discoverer of the circulatory system

April 26, 2:45 P.M.

I'm sitting in the acupuncturist's waiting room, comforted by a sweet, musky scent in the air and the sight of all sorts of interesting books and artifacts with an Eastern flavor. I've never liked needles; I hate getting shots and almost pass out half the time, but the good news is that I'm just interviewing her, so I can calm down. I'm hoping that she has a different perspective from the other doctors, because they're starting to get repetitive.

April 26, 3:05 P.M.

I'm now sitting on the acupuncture table. She wants to talk with me *and* give me a treatment. Yikes! She said a treatment is worth a thousand words, and I'll be able to feel the calming benefits rather than hear her explain them. I feel like such a chicken. I hope she knows what she's doing.

April 26, 4:30 P.M.

It's a beautiful afternoon, and I feel so relaxed. I decided to drive to a park to meditate. The sunlight is glistening on the leaves of the trees. I feel centered, emotionally sturdy, and comfortable in my own skin right now, and I want the feelings to sink in.

April 26, 4:50 P.M.

I fell asleep and had the sweetest dream: Mom was alive. Her blue-green eyes with specks of gold gazed straight into mine. I felt so connected and safe. I really miss her, but I'm breathing deeply, accepting the pain in my heart and the tears are streaming down my face. This is progress; ordinarily I would be mad at myself for feeling sad.

A car honking just disturbed the feeling, but I got it back. I was irritated, but then I closed my eyes and concentrated on the fresh scents of the greenery that filled me with a vibrant sensation.

The visit with the acupuncturist was interesting. First she checked my pulse and asked me how I'd been feeling. I told her that ever since Dad's heart attack I've been more anxious, irritable, and tired than usual. She told me my pulse sounded hollow, which indicated I might be directing a lot of energy outside and very little inside to nourish myself.

She said the energy in my heart and the strength in my blood is weak. She gave me a treatment to nourish the blood and heart centers and to redirect my energy to these areas. The needles didn't really hurt—just felt a little funny. She played soft, soothing music while I lay there with the needles in me. A warm, relaxed feeling came over me—a new, quiet feeling that's hard to describe. I feel calmer from deep inside.

She said (just as the others had) that emotional stability is important for preventing heart disease. Some people have more trouble handling emotional upset than others, especially if they feel they have to be in control all the time. I told her sometimes my heart feels as if it's flip-flopping. She also suggested I try meditation or yoga.

April 28, 8:30 P.M.

It's hard to describe, but I feel a little quieter inside. In one way I'm not like myself, but in another way I'm more like myself than I've ever been before.

I stopped by Dad's house the other day. I'm so happy he's home. He told me about his cardiac support group at the hospital. As he said before, they are supposed to talk about their personal lives, not their work. He said he talked about me!

He told everyone how proud he is of me and how important I am to him. They asked him if he tells me that, and he said "No," but he promised the group that he would tell me. He said he had always thought that what made him successful in life was his intense, tough, no-nonsense attitude, but he felt better about his marriage to Mom and raising me than about any other accomplishments. It blew me away to hear him talk like that, and I felt very special.

Doctor's Notepad

Lack of emotional stability puts stress on the cardiovascular system. The heart is not just an organ; it's an energy system that emotional turmoil and heartbreak can weaken. Emotional problems over a long period of time can lead to blood stagnation in the chest and energy deficiency in the heart. A protective layer of energy can develop around the heart and make it function sluggishly.

According to Chinese medicine, "The mind resides in the heart," so imbalance in the heart affects the mind, and imbalance in the mind affects the function of the heart. When the heart and the blood are healthy, they help the mind be strong, content, and calm. When the heart or blood functions weakly, the result can be mental agitation, irritability, depression, anxiety, insomnia, and generally low spirits. Once this kind of cycle has begun, it's best to approach it from all sides: physical, mental, and spiritual.

Let's take relationships, for instance. The mind and heart relate closely to each other in responses to life experience and in the capacity for love. If a person feels hurt in his heart about a relationship, his mind is unlikely to be at peace about love, and if a person is in an agitated mental state, his heart cannot be energized by love. To have stable, loving relationships, one must have a certain amount of internal balance between these functions.

The most important thing you should do after a heart attack is to reevaluate what's important in your life. If you had a heart attack, something in your life was seriously off balance. We need to learn how to live with ourselves peacefully. The practice of compassion and forgiveness can be a powerful antidote to anger. Compassion can be defined as unconditional acceptance and understanding with a desire to alleviate one's suffering (self or other). Practicing compassion and forgiveness with ourselves can soften the harsh inner critic in our minds.

Practicing compassion and forgiveness toward others can soothe our heart's energy and help us heal our relationships. Many tools are available to help balance energy. Qi gong, tai chi, and yoga are excellent methods for practicing breathing, concentration, and movements that can improve your physical, mental, emotional, and spiritual health. When the human system is clear and its energy unrestricted, the immune system is empowered, and emotional stability and mental clarity are elevated. Acupuncture can also help re-balance one's energy after open heart surgery and other traumatic heart incidents.

Chapter Nine

The Recovered Person:
Healing Your Relationships

"Before sunlight can shine through a window, the blinds must be raised."

—American Proverb

May 1, 11:30 P.M.

I had a great time having dinner with David, Dr. James's friend, and his wife and two kids. We had grilled halibut, wild rice, wheat berries, and steamed veggies. I didn't know that healthy food could taste so good.

The people were warm and nice. I felt welcome, yet they claimed their household used to be very tense and stressed. After his first heart attack David changed his diet and started to exercise more regularly. Then he had a second one, and got really scared. He said that after the first one he didn't think he needed the cardiac rehab program and didn't have time for it. He always resented anyone telling him what to do. The second time, he decided to follow all the advice his medical team gave him.

He decreased his work hours as an emergency-room doctor and found that he liked meditation, and enjoyed the classes where he learned more about what made him tick. Like me, he found a place of peace inside himself. He practices going there during meditations and says it gets easier to access the more he tries. He also learned a lot about himself in counseling and began to reorganize his priorities. Maybe I could use counseling…

David says he got in touch with how hard he is on himself and started to practice all kinds of relaxation exercises. He read books and chose what felt most natural for him. I like him, and I'm really glad he's still here to talk about his experiences. He said each day is precious. Before, his life was flying by and he was missing the important parts, but now he feels as if he's present in each moment.

He used to be a workaholic and didn't even know that he was miserable. Work was the only thing that made him feel worthwhile, but he was tired, angry, and resentful of everyone around him. His kids said he used to be a control freak and a perfectionist who drove them all crazy, but he's gotten better. His whole family said they have a lot more fun with him now, and his oldest son whispered to me that his dad is "more human" now.

After dinner David and I went for a walk in their avocado groves. He admitted to me that he used to blame every one but himself for his problems. His recent studies have taught him that his experiences in life are determined largely by his thoughts. When he had fearful thoughts he created negativity in his environment; when he had a compassionate perspective, he experienced more love. Having a heart attack, he said, can bring your whole life into perspective.

I feel dizzy as I realize the amount of responsibility I have for my own well-being and quality of life. David asked me how anyone can know God without spending time with God. He spends twenty minutes a day with God. First he spills his guts out loud for five minutes or so, telling Him everything that is on his mind. Then he tells God everything that he is grateful for, and then he is quiet and listens to God. He said that these twenty minutes a day have changed his life.

May 2, 7:30 A.M.

I feel inspired by David. I spent a few minutes being quiet, breathing, listening within, and feeling good! If I stop doing the breathing exercises, even for a few days, I have a hard time getting started again. I was always taught that I should be doing, doing, doing, so quieting my mind goes against everything I've ever learned.

May 2, 3:00 P.M.

I had a tense moment at work, feeling frustrated with customers and my assistant at the same time. I need to work on my temper and my communication skills. David said his recovery involved learning to communicate better with people, especially his wife and kids. He wasn't really listening to people, but telling them what to do and expecting them to obey him. He said he and his wife are much closer now.

May 2, 10:00 P.M.

I just finished reading a beautiful book, The Miracle of Mindfulness, by That Nhat Han. I'm more productive and less tired when I try to go through my day mindfully. I also feel calmer.

May 3, 10:00 P.M.

I'm feeling impatient with myself. I learn this stuff that helps, and still can't do it all the time. I guess it takes practice. I think of what David said about living my life as if each moment were my last. When I try to get into that perspective I feel amazingly calm, almost relaxed.

David said the most important part of his recovery was gaining the love and support of his family by reducing his workload and spending more quality time with them. He even started to enjoy his work more when he was there. He practices learning to flow with life, instead of trying to make everything into the shape he thinks it should be. Taking time for reflection and quiet helps him get perspective so he doesn't get as worked up over little things.

I was embarrassed, but I asked David anyway, "How can a person become more loving?"

He said it starts with loving and appreciating oneself. Why don't I? I think one of the things that drive me is hoping that someday Dad will be proud of me. Even though he said the other day that he was proud of me, I still feel he has incredibly high standards for me, and I'll never quite measure up. He'll keep raising the bar. I wish it weren't so important to me. I wish I didn't feel so self-conscious around him. I need to work on feeling better about myself, no matter what anyone else thinks.

David believes what people need most from each other is "the gift of their loving presence." He told me I should forgive Dad for disappointing me and just give him my loving presence.

He took me through an exercise where I put my hand over my heart and relax while paying attention to my breathing. At first I felt tightness and fear in my gut. I kept breathing, slowly and deeply; the tightness softened, and an ache replaced it. Then David told me to try to forgive the hurts Dad has caused me and to focus on my feelings of love for him. I felt the ache around my heart lift.

He said that if I practice slowing down and centering myself on the loving feeling in my heart I'll increase my capacity to love. When I'm with Dad I should focus on the love I feel for him, be grateful that he's here, and tell myself that my love is important to him.

May 3, 1:00 A.M.

I couldn't sleep, kept tossing and turning. I was mad at myself for not being further along in every area of my life, and I felt nervous. I must try an exercise that David showed me.

May 4, 1:20 A.M.

I did breathing exercises, and when I was relaxed I imagined myself in one of my favorite places up in the mountains. I could feel the sun on my skin and the crisp breeze in the air. The sky was blue, clean, and clear. I could see patches of thin snow still melting from the winter, and delicate, determined little wildflowers blooming here and there. David said to wait till a particular image called to me and then talk to it, so I talked to the little yellow daisies.

I said "Hello," told them how beautiful their home was, and said how much I appreciated them. Then I apologized to them for disturbing their peace, and the daisies told me that it was nice to have me there. I suddenly became aware of feeling worthless, and I shared that with the daisies. They said, "You're alive. Anything that is part of life is beautiful." That touched me, and I felt a sense of calm and vitality when I finished the exercise. I must remember this.

Doctor's Notepad

David changed his dietary, exercise, and work habits after his first heart attack, but only after his second heart attack did he seriously reevaluate his attitudes, emotions, thoughts, and priorities. He then reorganized his work life and changed his thinking in many ways. He learned to meditate, relax, spend time with God, and develop closer, more loving relationships with his family. He feels happier and healthier than he ever has before.

Alice is beginning to apply some of what she is learning to her daily life. She has started to practice breathing, relaxation, and meditation exercises. She experiments with guided imagery by taking herself in her mind to a beautiful, safe place and allowing herself to interact with an image that she feels drawn toward. Alice demonstrates how guided imagery can stimulate our healer within. When she spends a morning with her father, they enjoy seeing how they have each grown as a result of his heart attack, and they appreciate their loving connection.

Meditation is referred to throughout this book. There are many different methods of meditation. Religious traditions such as Judaism, Christianity, Catholicism, and Islam, and philosophies such as Buddhism and Taoism have different systems for meditation. Explore various methods and stay with the ones you find most effective. Any effort you make toward becoming more self-aware can be helpful. Breathe deeply while you read inspirational material.

Good communication skills are essential for healthy relationships. People need to feel safe to tell those they love how they really feel. This is especially challenging for CPBP folks; among this group, men generally find it even more difficult to speak with their loved ones about their true feelings. Many boys are taught that only girls cry, and it can be very difficult to change this training, but disclosing your true feelings to those close to you is good for your heart's health and will improve your relationships.

The tendency to blame other people for your negative feelings and experiences is common in human nature. You must resist the "blame game" and take responsibility for your thoughts and attitudes and behavior that contribute to the situations and experiences in which you find yourselves.

Some suggestions for improving your relationships (with yourself and others):

1. Spend a minimum of twenty minutes a day in some type of meditation. Pick the one that works best for you. Twenty minutes a day in conscious contact with your own spiritual or philosophical connection to "the universe"—God as you understand God—is recommended. Don't do any other activities simultaneously; just focus on getting to know this connectedness and letting it get to know you.

2. When communicating with an angry person, empathize with them instead of defending yourself, e.g. "I understand that you are frustrated and don't want me to be late anymore." Do your best to listen compassionately with all your heart.

3. When expressing anger yourself, try to use words like "I feel" or "I'm experiencing or observing," rather than starting your communication with "you." You will be less likely to put the other person on the defense.

4. Try to understand the suffering of the people you love. Understanding them deeply can help you take the actions toward that person that will help them feel happy and loved.

Chapter Ten

The Father and Daughter: A Moment of Grace

"We are all connected by a membrane of light. The Kabbalahist believe that when you are in a healthy relationship, the light is not obstructed."

—A Kabbalahist perspective shared by Gail Gross, Ph.D.

May 5, 3:00 P.M.

I went to bed early last night, after doing a progressive muscle relaxation exercise I found in a book. I tightened my toes and feet for thirty seconds and then relaxed them, tightened my legs for thirty seconds and relaxed them, and so on up my body to my hands, squeezing my fists tightly for thirty seconds and releasing them, then my face. This stuff really works; I slept like a baby. I wanted to be rested for my visit with Dad today.

I spent the whole morning with him. We took a beautiful walk. He seems softer and calmer, and said he likes the cardiac rehab program at the hospital. It was nice to walk and talk with him. I told him what I've been learning, and he recognized that I'm in a good place.

We talked about how beautiful the day was, with billowy white clouds against a backdrop of blue sky and the apricot trees with their delicate new buds. The moon and the sun were sharing the sky at opposite ends of the horizon. Dad and I walked along, enjoying just being together. I felt more relaxed with him than I've ever been. I didn't push him to talk about how he's feeling, just hung out with him, and it was great. I can hardly believe it happened.

At one point Dad took my hand and held it for a while as we walked. I told him how glad I was that he's here. He squeezed my hand and told me that he loved me. I really felt he did.

Doctor's Notepad

The reward for choosing more positive thoughts and behaviors can be a healthier body, mind, spirit, and overall quality of life.

The Coronary-Prone Behavior Pattern is a rushed and chronically hostile approach to life.

Hostility can be very destructive to your health and relationships. Hostile people tend to more isolated, lonely, and depressed. The best relationship include being able to talk about negative feelings without hostility. If you feel poor physically, emotionally, or spiritually, look to your own behavior: diet, exercise, sleep, water consumption, thoughts, and relationships. It is common (especially, it seems, among people with C.P.B.P.) to blame external situations and people for our negative feelings. The "blame game" can make us feel trapped in circumstances that seem beyond our control. If you feel that you can't get a grip on self-destructive behaviors, consult a professional for assistance. We all need help from time to time. We human beings are social creatures. We need one another for companionship, compassion, love, and partnership of different types; this may be with your spouse, your physician, or the person who comes regularly to pick up our garbage. We might have less heart disease if we cultivated a more compassionate attitude toward all humanity, individually and collectively—beginning with ourselves.

Understanding your own tendencies toward the coronary-prone behavior Pattern can help you begin to make changes. The most important aspects of CPBP are time urgency and chronic hostility or irritability. Anger management and time management can be very helpful. Once you understand the coronary prone behavior pattern and how destructive it can be, you can start using this book to guide you in making changes to improve your health.

The truth is that we have very limited control in the world. Inner strength, character, and optimal health involve taking responsibility for ourselves and trying to make the best of our lives. It is what we do with our experiences and how we choose to behave that determines the quality of individual and collective quality of life.

Changing the way you relate to life, yourself, and other people is important in reducing your risk of cardiovascular illness. You can make the changes suggested in this book to improve your life.

References

Allan, Robert, Ph.D., and Stephen Scheidt, M.D., *Heart and Mind: The Practice of Cardiac Psychology*. American Psychological Association, 1996.

Anderson, Norman, Ph.D., Director of NIH's Office of Behavior and Social Research: The Impact of Stress on Health: Recent findings from NIH-F.

Bair, Puran. *Living From the Heart, Heart Rhythm Meditation for Energy, Clarity, Peace, Joy and Inner Power*. New York: Random House, 1998.

Brahe, Carl. *Healing on the Edge of Now, A Practical Guide for the Use of Psychoneuroimmunology*. Colorado: Press Publications, 1992.

Chang, P. et al, "*Anger in Young Men and Subsequent Premature Cardiovascular Disease: The Precursors Study*," Archives of Internal Medicine; 162 (8):901-6. Apr. 22, 2002.

Charlesworth, Edward, A., Ph.D. *Stress Management: A Comprehensive Guide to Wellness*. Biobehavioral Press, 1982.

Chodron, Pema. *Awakening Loving Kindness*. Shambhala Pocket Classics. December, 1996.

Cousins, Norman. *The Healing Heart; Antidotes to Panic and Helplessness.* New York, London: W.W. Norton and Company, 1983.

Dali Lama and Vreeland. *An Open Heart: Practicing Compassion in Everyday Life.* Little Brown and Company; 1st ed. September 25, 2001.

Dali Lama and Cutler. *The Art of Happiness; A Handbook for Living.* Riverhead Books; November, 1998.

Davis, Martha, Ph.D., Eshelman, Elizabeth Robbins, M.S.W., McKay, Matthew, Ph.D., *The Relaxation and Stress Reduction Workbook,* 5th Ed., New Harbinger Publications, Inc. Oakland, Ca., 2000

Farhi, Donna. *The Breathing Book.* Holt. 1996.

Friedman, Howard, S., *Hostility, Coping and Health.* American Psychological Association, 1992.

Glaser, Ronald, and Janice Glaser-Kiecolt. *Human Stress and Immunity.* Academic Press, Inc., 1994

Hanh, Thich Nhat. *The Miracle of Mindfulness.* Boston: Beacon Press, 1987.

Hanh, Thich Nhat. *Anger: Wisdom for Cooling the Flames.* Riverhead Books, NY.NY. 2001.

Institute of Science, Technology and Public Policy, Fairfield, IA, 52557. Ornish, D.M., M.D., *Cardiovascular Risk Factors* (July 1992) 276-280

Kabat-Zinn, Jon, Ph.D. *Full Catastrophe Living.* New York, New York: Dell Publishing, 1990.

Kornfield, Jack. *The Art of Forgiveness, Lovingkindness and Peace.* Bantam Books. August, 2002.

Lipsenthal, Lee, M.D. Medical Director, Preventive Medicine Research Institute. (Dean Ornish, M.D.) : *Behavioral and Physiological Benefits of Stress Management in Treatment of Coronary Artery Disease.*

Marks, William, E. *The Holy Order of Water, Healing Earth's Waters and Ourselves*, Bell Pond Books, Great Barrington, MA. 01230, 2001 Maximin, Anita, Psy.D. Lori Stevic-Rust, Ph.D., Lori White Kenyon, Ph.D. *Heart Therapy, Regaining Your Cardiac Health.* California: New Harbinger Publications, 1997.

Milkman, Dan. *No Ordinary Moments.* California: H.J. Kramer, Inc., 1992.

Michel, Judith, Dr., and Dr. Shalom Srebrenica. *Beyond Your Ego.* C.I.S. Publishers and Distributors, International. 1991.

Meyers, Bill. *Healing and the Mind.* New York: Doubleday, 1993.

Newman, James, W, Release Your Brakes, 2[nod] Edition, *the Pace Organization*, Del Mar, California, 2001.

Ornish, Dean, M.D. *Love and Survival.* New York, New York: HarperCollins Publishing, 1997.

Ornish, Dean, M.D. *Stress, Diet and Your Heart*. New York: Holt, Rinehart and Winston, 1982.

Myss, Caroline, Ph.D., and C. Norman Shealy, M.D., Ph.D. *The Creation of Health*. New York, New York: Three Rivers Press, 1988.

Ojeda, Linda, Ph.D., *Her Healthy Heart*, Hunter House Inc., Alameda, California, 1998.

Pearsall, Paul, Ph.D. *The Heart's Code, the New Findings about Cellular Memories and Their Role in the Mind/Body/Spirit Connection*. New York: Broadway Books, 1999.

Pliskin, Zelig. *Gateway to Happiness*. The Jewish Learning Exchange, 1983.

Rinpoche, Sogyal *The Tibetan Book of Living and Dying*. New York, New York: HarperCollins Publishers, Inc., 1994.

Rosenberg, Marshall, B. PhD. *Nonviolent Communication, A Language of Compassion*. Puddle Dancer Press, Encinitas, CA.92023-1129.

Rossi Lawrence, Ernest. *The Psychobiology of Mind-Body Healing*. New York, London: W.W. Norton and Company, Inc., 1986.

Schiffman, Erich. *Yoga, the Spirit and Practice of Moving into Stillness*. New York: Pocket Books, 1996.

Schneider, R.H., et al., *Hypertension* 26 (1995) 820-827) and 28 (1996) 228-248.

Stoney, C., Ph.D., Ohio State University. *Life Sciences Journal,* May 14, 1999. Study supported part by the <u>National Institutes of Health</u> and Ohio State's General Clinical Research Center.

Toole, Eckhart. *The Power of Now.* New World Library, Novato, CA, 1999.

Weil, Andrew, M.D. *Eight Weeks to Optimum Health.* Alfred A. Knopf, Inc. 1997.

Weil, Andrew, M.D. *Spontaneous Healing.* New York: Knopf. 1995.

About the Author

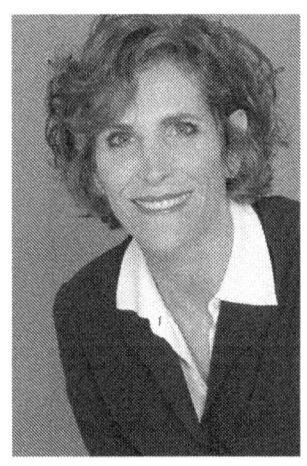

Diana Wisdom Ph.D., is a licensed clinical psychologist (psy# 12476) in private practice in Del Mar, California. She is married and has three step-daughters. She specializes in cardiac psychology, stress management, optimal health, and productivity. She is an educational and inspirational speaker. Through years of research and practical application, Dr. Wisdom has established gentle, effective methods for reprogramming oneself to reduce the incidence of heart attack and heart disease.

The author may be contacted at:

The Del Mar Clinic
240 9th Street
Del Mar, California, 92014
(858) 259 0146
www.drdianawisdom.com

www.ingramcontent.com/pod-product-compliance
Lightning Source LLC
Chambersburg PA
CBHW020258290526
45784CB00003B/1285